Penguin Books

Make it Happy, Make it Safe

Jane Cousins-Mills (previously Cousins) was born in London in 1948, and read History at the University of Kent. She worked as researcher for Martin Gilbert, Churchill's biographer, and then as research assistant to Sir Harold Wilson. From 1973 to 1975 she was with Granada Television's 'World in Action' team and was a reporter-presenter on Granada's daily local news programme. She has been secretary to the Sexual Law Reform Society and to the Defence of Literature and the Arts Society. She was Director of the Edinburgh International Television Festival from 1977 to 1979. Her interest in sex education led her to working with teenagers, their parents and teachers on the subject and to presenting a weekly sex phone-in programme for Manchester's Piccadilly Radio. From 1984 to 1986 she was Head of Production at the National Film and Television School. At present she is an independent film-maker and writer, Chairperson of the Executive Committee of the Edinburgh Television Festival and Vice-Chairperson of the Edinburgh International Film Festival. Her books include *Turkey! Torture and Political Persecution* (1973), the highly successful *Make it Happy* (1980), winner of *The Times Educational Supplement* Senior Information Book Award, and *Womanwords* (1988).

JANE COUSINS-MILLS

Make it Happy, Make it Safe

WHAT SEX IS ALL ABOUT

PENGUIN BOOKS

PENGUIN BOOKS

Published by the Penguin Group
27 Wrights Lane, London W8 5TZ, England
Viking Penguin Inc., 40 West 23rd Street, New York, New York 10010, USA
Penguin Books Australia Ltd, Ringwood, Victoria, Australia
Penguin Books Canada Ltd, 2801 John Street, Markham, Ontario, Canada L3R 1B4
Penguin Books (NZ) Ltd, 182–190 Wairau Road, Auckland 10, New Zealand

Penguin Books Ltd, Registered Offices: Harmondsworth, Middlesex, England

First published by Virago, under the title Make it Happy, 1978
Second edition 1979
Published in Penguin Books 1980
Reprinted with revisions 1986
Third edition, under the title Make it Happy, Make it Safe, 1988

Copyright © Jane Cousins-Mills, 1978, 1979, 1986, 1988
Drawings copyright © Audrey Besterman, 1988
Photographs on pages 24, 106, 109, 111, 114, 117, 121
copyright © Maggie Murray, 1988
All rights reserved

Made and printed in Great Britain by
Cox and Wyman Ltd, Reading, Berks.
Filmset in Trump Mediaeval by
Rowland Phototypesetting Ltd, Bury St Edmunds, Suffolk

Contents

7 The Misuse and Abuse of Sex   81

Incest and abuse of care, telling · Rape: if you are raped – some guidelines, do you report a rape?; reporting it to the police; getting over the rape · Dirty phone calls · Flashers · Peeping Toms · Sexual harassment · Pornography · Prostitution · Prevention: some dos and don'ts

8 Birth Control   99

The myths · Whose responsibility? Legal position · Where to get contraception · Live in the Republic of Ireland? Reliable methods: the pill, the mini-pill, the morning-after pill, the coil, the morning-after coil; the condom, the cap; spermicides; injectables; sterilization · Unreliable methods: natural methods; withdrawal, holding back, douche, sponge

9 Pregnancy   128

How to tell · Pregnancy testing · If you're not pregnant · If you are pregnant · First reactions · Who to tell

10 Abortion   135

How safe? How to get an abortion: if you are under 16; getting a free abortion on the National Health Service; private or charitable abortion services, commercial abortion services, live in Northern Ireland?, live in the Republic of Ireland? · Methods of abortion · After the abortion

11 Having a Baby   143

Where to stay · Leaving home · Medical care · Finding out about pregnancy and childbirth · Living together · Marriage · Adoption and fostering · Education · Work · Money · Rights of the father · Maintenance

12 Make it Healthy   152

Prevention of disease · General symptoms · Where to get treatment: at the clinic · Contact tracing · Illnesses and sexually transmitted diseases: AIDS, candida albicans (thrush), cancers, chlamydia; cystitis; gardnerella; gonorrhoea; hepatitis; herpes; lice; menstrual problems; pelvic inflammatory disease; scabies; syphilis; trichomoniasis; urethritis; warts

Acknowledgements

Although this book is a re-write rather than an updated and revised edition of the original, I would like to thank all those who helped me then and with intervening revised versions: Rose Ades, Pam Adshead, Margaret Branch, the Brook Advisory Centre, the Campaign for Homosexual Equality, Taransay Chisholm, Shirley Clarke, Cathy Crawford, Bobbie Crosby, Roy Cuthbert, Nick Free, Tess Gill, Judy Gray, Bob Greaves, Jim Greaves, Antony Grey, Gail Hamilton, Pat Hawes, Mike Jarvis, Sylvia Jones, Nina Kellgren, Charles Kitchen, Thelma McGough, Pete Mackertitch, Jonathon Lawton, Jill Liddington, Trevor Locke, London Gay Switchboard, Lorraine, Joyce Mastin, Diane Mundy, the National Council for One Parent Families, Ursula Owen, Pam Peart, Angela Phillips, Michael Rubinstein, Eleanor Rubinstein, Eleanor Stephens, Ruth Stockley, Kate Swan, the Terrence Higgins Trust, Virago Press, the Women's National Cancer Control Campaign, and Lynne Wright.

For the work done on this book I give special thanks to Sandra Ferguson for all her excellent and really thorough research. Once again the Campaign for Homosexual Equality and the Terrence Higgins Trust were wonderfully helpful, as were London Gay Switchboard. Others who have helped me and whom I wish to thank are Clara, Chris, the Irish Family Planning Association, Jessica, Melanie MacFadyean, Sadie, Müjde Ar and Tina Wiseman.

I am particularly grateful to Audrey Besterman for her drawings on pages 12, 16, 17, 20, 28, 71, 115, 118 and 169, which I consider to be very fine indeed. My thanks, too, to Maggie Murray, who took the photographs on pages 24, 105, 109, 110, 111, 114, 116, 117, 121. Further thanks are due to the B Team Resources for Boys Work poster on page 33, Joanne O'Brien Format for the photograph on page 38, Cath Jackson for the cartoon on page 65, the Health Education Authority for the poster on page 101, Board of Health, Guernsey/Family Planning Sales of Oxford for the cartoons on page 161 and the Albany Trust Sex Education Project, Deptford, for the poster on page 176. Pam Dix, my editor, was consistently helpful, sympathetic and a great pleasure to work with. Also at Penguin I should like to thank Lynne Bruce and Judy Gordon. I am very grateful to Ronnie Fraser for reading and making invaluable comments on the manuscript. To Elaine Steel I offer my sincere thanks for her toughness and friendship.

Finally, I would like to thank Lady Forman who, sadly, died while I was writing this book. Her perceptive comments and criticisms about the first version were never far from my mind as I wrote. She would have enjoyed knowing that she finally won the argument.

J. C.-M.

CHAPTER ONE

Making it Happy and Safe

This book used to be called simply *Make it Happy*. I wrote it back in the late 1970s because it seemed to me that not enough young people knew very much about how their bodies worked or about what was happening to them when they had sexual feelings or relationships. Even more tricky, sometimes, is working out the connections between our feelings of respect, affection or love for someone and our sexual feelings.

My main aim was to help those who found it difficult to talk with their parents, teachers, friends or someone who really knew about these things. No one knows everything there is to know about sex, but it struck me that the less we know, the more likely we are to make some sort of unnecessary mistake. Everyone makes some mistake or other when it comes to thinking about, or having, a sexual relationship. They're not always very serious, but for some they are. I didn't think anyone should make a mistake or have a problem just because they don't know the facts. So, after talking to scores of teenagers (and their parents, teachers, social workers, doctors, etc.), what I did was to write a book which showed how you could avoid certain problems which were caused simply by not knowing, not understanding or having no one to ask.

For those who found themselves with a really big problem, I wanted to help them understand that there are ways of solving it. Lots of help organizations exist for you: there isn't a single problem that loads of others haven't had to face at some time or other.

You'll notice that this book has got a slightly different title. I've added *Make it Safe* to it. I've done this because several things have changed. The most obvious one is the disease called AIDS (which stands for Acquired Immune Deficiency Syndrome). Before, most problems were either solvable or at least possible to cope with. Sadly, this isn't the case any longer because AIDS can kill and there isn't yet a cure.

But you can prevent AIDS. One of the reasons that people get AIDS is that they don't have safer sex. Some people don't know about safer sex. Others know about it in theory but not when it comes down to practice. Many governments all round the world have launched 'Don't die of ignorance' type campaigns. But when we're scared of something – and who isn't scared of dying? – we either don't learn properly or we take risks, hoping and pretending to ourselves that it won't happen to us.

People take crazy risks all the time even though they know what they're doing is dangerous. It's like people who drink and drive. It's too late after there's been an accident for the drunk driver to wonder why they didn't walk or take a taxi rather than take the car. An awful lot of people of all ages don't practise safer sex even though they know they should. It's not just daft; it's much more serious than that because AIDS is the one sexually transmitted disease that can and does kill. You can't cure it – you have to prevent it.

It's important for everyone to know about safer sex, not just those who are already having a sex life. There's a lot of wrong information around both about sex and about AIDS. And there are some people who use the subject of AIDS to try to make young people feel scared, guilty or ashamed about their sexual feelings. It really is nonsense to say that AIDS proves that sex before marriage or with more than one partner is sinful. And it's not a disease that only homosexuals (people who are sexually attracted to people of the same sex as themselves) get.

I think there's room for a whole range of views about sex

and that people should do what they think is right for them. But I don't think it's at all OK for anyone to try to force everyone else to have exactly the same views. Nor is it OK to use AIDS as an excuse for making us feel guilty, scared or ashamed about our sexual feelings. Because this is exactly what makes us want to bury our heads in the sand and stay ignorant rather than take informed decisions about our own lives. And we all ought to realize that we should spend our time and energy attacking disease and illness rather than attacking people who want to have a love life.

I believe that ignorance causes a lot of harm but that knowledge and information don't. That's why this book is written not only for those who are already having a sexual relationship but also for those who are just wondering what it's all about. If you want to know the answer to a question, then you're ready for the answer.

In many ways I think it would be great if this book – or any other book like it – didn't have to be written. If parents, teachers and other adults knew the answers to all our questions and realized that wanting to know about sex was a natural part of being a human being, then there wouldn't be a need for any book. But many adults don't know all the answers, lots of us grow up without a parent to turn to, and teachers – like all adults – can also feel quite uptight when talking about sex. Just look at the advice pages in newspapers and magazines aimed at adults – the questions are often just the same as those you see in a teen mag.

I'm sad that this book has to start off with mentioning some of the bad-news aspects of sex. Sex, whether we're thinking about it and asking questions or whether we're involved in a sexual relationship, isn't only about the dangers and problems.

Probably one of the most important things to learn about sex is that it's a healthy and natural part of our lives. This doesn't mean that everyone has to have an active sex life. Some people find that sex is a big part of their lives, others prefer life with very little sex or none at all. And people have sex for a variety of different reasons. It can be because they're curious, because it seems like a good way of expressing friendship and affection, because they want some fun or because they're in love. But you can also be friendly, have fun or be in love and not have sex. Each one of us has different sexual feelings and needs and these can change and vary throughout our lives. There are lots of different reasons why people don't want a sexual relationship. It may be that they're not in love or simply because they don't feel like it.

Love is a complicated subject. Lots of grown-ups think that when you're young you can't be in love. In the end no one can easily tell you what your own feelings are. Only you can work that out. When you are in love it's only natural to want to share your innermost feelings with your partner. And wanting to show your love sexually is natural too. Sex, like love, isn't just about getting pleasure – it's also about giving pleasure. This means treating your partner honestly, truthfully, fairly, equally and lovingly.

It never makes sense to lie to anyone about your feelings. Sometimes people feel under pressure to have sex when they don't really want to. Or you might feel that if your boyfriend or girlfriend really loved you then they would agree to go to bed with you. But trying to persuade someone to have sex – or, worse still, trying to force them by putting heavy pressure on them – isn't about love. It's about power. And it's about treating someone like a bit of dirt. Telling someone you love them simply in order to persuade them to have sex with you is not only dishonest, it can also be harmful. It will make them feel used and could prevent them from feeling good about sex for the rest of their lives.

Love and sex are connected – but they're also separate at the same time. Working out just how they're connected and how they're separate can be tricky. You might be very much in love with someone but feel very scared about your sexual feelings. No advice column, no book, can solve everyone's problems but there are a lot of people who could solve their own problems if only they had a bit more information. Sex can, and does, make a lot of people very happy.

This book will give you some of the basic information

about sex, and will tell you how some of the problems can be avoided and where to go if you need more help or advice. It's written for teenagers (and their parents, teachers and anyone else) who want to learn about the basic facts. Girls and boys who want to find out what sex might be about when they're older, and also older people who still aren't quite sure, may be able to learn from this book how they can safely ignore many of the myths and incorrect information about sex which often make it all unnecessarily complicated.

Safer sex is just one side of avoiding certain problems that can arise when two people start having a sexual relationship. Just as important is how you feel towards someone and how you treat them. It seems to me to be a good idea always to treat someone as you would like to be treated yourself. That's the only way to make it really happy.

CHAPTER TWO

Minds and Bodies

Though it's obviously a bit hard to prove, our sex lives probably start even before we're born. It's known for certain that many boys are born with an erect penis, and although it's not so easy to tell when girls first show signs of being sexually active, there's no reason to suppose it's any later than it is for boys.

From birth onwards a lot is known about our sex lives. Both girls and boys can reach a peak of sexual excitement before they're six months old, and most of us, although by no means all, touch our sex organs for the pleasure of it throughout our childhood. Many of the games small children play are very sexual. Games like 'doctors' and 'mothers and fathers' often end up with kids getting and giving each other good sexual feelings. Literally millions of kids over the ages have played these games without coming to the slightest harm. It's a different matter, of course, if an older child or even an adult either forces a child or somehow makes a child experiment in this way. But many parents are convinced that even the harmless sort of game is wrong or dangerous and try to stop their children from touching themselves where it feels nice.

Sex is a natural part of our lives, whatever our age. A slap on the hand to stop us from touching our sex organs, or genitals as they're also called, when we're young can cause a lot of harm because it makes us grow up feeling guilty or scared of our bodies and of our sexual feelings. It can make us grow up thinking that sex must be wrong and in some way dirty. In fact touching ourselves, finding out how our bodies look and work sexually, and getting sexual feelings, can't do us any harm. And growing up feeling guilty, ashamed or scared of sex doesn't do us any good at all.

Puberty, adolescence, maturity

Throughout childhood the genitals we were born with stay more or less the same. A girl has a clitoris, a vagina and inside her body a uterus, or womb, and two ovaries. A boy has a penis, two testicles that are usually called balls, and inside he has all his internal organs too.

But as we get to being a teenager our body starts to produce natural chemicals called hormones, which alter its shape and appearance and which make our sex organs become sexually mature. This process is called puberty. For a girl, the first sign that she's beginning to mature is when her breasts start to develop. Hair grows around her genitals and under her arms. Her genitals go a darker, more reddish colour of pink, become more fleshy and more sensitive to touch. For a boy, it's when pubic hairs start to grow around the base of his penis. His testicles will also have started to develop, but at first this isn't usually very noticeable. Hair grows around the base of his penis, under his arms and eventually – although usually not until he's sixteen or older – on his face and perhaps on his chest. After a bit of wavering and squeaking, his voice breaks and goes much deeper.

Very often, while the production of these hormones is getting properly balanced, the skin can get very greasy and we get a spotty complexion. Some people get spots on their backs as well. It helps to eat fresh vegetables and fruit, lean meat and fish, and to keep off puddings, butter, milk, eggs and sweets. You can buy creams and medicated soap from the chemist which help clear up the spots or, if they're really bad, your doctor should be able to prescribe some extra-strong cream. Spots, pimples and blackheads will disappear in time – squeezing and picking them only makes them worse and may leave you with a pitted skin. It isn't easy, but try to leave them alone.

You may find that you suddenly start to sweat very heavily. Clean sweat doesn't smell bad, but if it's left on your body it can soon start to smell unpleasant. Washing well once or twice a day with a medicated soap helps to prevent the smell probably better than roll-on, spray or aerosol deodorants. Many of these try to mask the smell instead of killing the bacteria on the skin which produce the smell.

All these changes can be quite scary – especially if they happen quite fast. Older people and younger sisters and brothers often find it annoyingly funny to see the changes take place and this can make many young people feel very embarrassed indeed about the fact that, for example, their breasts are developing or that their voice seems uncontrollable. All you can do is grit your teeth and bear it – there's nothing you can do to stop the changes from taking place.

The stage at which we reach maturity is when our sex organs have ripened or developed to the point at which it is technically possible for a girl or boy to have a baby. It's impossible to say exactly when this will happen – no two people ever reach puberty at exactly the same age. On average girls become sexually mature about two years before boys. The average age for girls is about 11 to 13 and for boys it's about 12 to 14. But this is only the average and it can happen as early as 9 or 10, or as late as 17 or 18. No one really knows why some of us are early developers and why others are late developers. It is known that those who have a healthy, balanced diet tend to develop earlier than those who don't. But mostly it's to do with the sort of body we inherited from our parents – and there's nothing we can do to alter that.

We can't control how long it takes for our bodies to mature either. At first our hormones are produced only rather irregularly. It takes time for them to be produced on a steady, balanced and regular basis. Some of us become physically and sexually mature very quickly; for others it can take several years.

After puberty comes adolescence. This means growing up mentally and emotionally. But the expression 'grown up' can mean different things to different people. We're often made to think that we have 'grown up' long before we really feel like it. Most adolescents – and so-called grown-ups, come to that – are a mixture of child and adult. You might find yourself feeling incredibly cool and sophisticated in one part of you, and yet still want to hug that old teddy bear at night. Maybe one of the reasons that adolescents get such a bad name for being confused or all over the place is that adults tend to be a bit better at hiding the child part of themselves from the rest of the world. But it is true that just as our hormones take time to settle down, so our thoughts, feelings and emotions take time to sort themselves out too.

Some teenagers find themselves falling in and out of love all the time. We often get crushes or strong feelings of sexual attraction and desire for someone of the same or opposite sex. It might be a crush on an older girl or boy at school, a teacher, a pop star, a footballer or a friend. Often these feelings fade away after a few weeks or months, but at the time it's not so easy to work out the difference between a sudden short crush and a deeper, stronger, perhaps more lasting, feeling of love. When it first happens to us it can all be rather bewildering. It's usually easier to understand what's happening to us by the time we've fallen for our third, fourth or fifth pop singer. But when you know, or think you know, that you're in love, it doesn't exactly help to be told that 'You'll grow out of it', or 'It's just a phase you're going through.' It doesn't feel like that at the time. And just as you might grow out of it, there's always a chance that you won't.

Any confusion we might feel at this time in our lives isn't helped much by the attitude of society towards sex. On the one hand adults seem to expect young people to behave as if they had no sexual feelings at all. And on the other, adults encourage teenagers to spend their money on clothes, make-up, magazines, etc., all designed to make them less childlike and more obviously sexually attractive. Teachers and parents spend a lot of time teaching kids to grow up – they teach us to read and write, cross roads safely and generally copy adult behaviour. But they don't always teach us very much about our sexual feelings. One teenage boy put it like this: 'My parents must have done it or I wouldn't have been born. But if they do it, how come they tell me it's dirty to even think about it?' It's not surprising that when we do eventually become aware of our sexual feelings, relationships can seem a bit complicated.

If life and relationships seem depressingly confused it may be worth remembering that almost everyone, whatever their age, makes the same sort of mistakes. To a large extent this confusion is caused by the sort of world we live in: we're encouraged to act, dress and think as if sex was ultra exciting, yet we're discouraged from acting on our sexual feelings. It's like getting the green light and the red light at the same time.

What we do, how we do it, with whom we do it, and how we feel about what we think and do is up to each one of us.

What we look like – girls

Breasts: Slang words for women's breasts include tits, titties, knockers and boobs. Most of the breast is made of fat. The rest consists of glands that produce milk after a baby is born, and tubes that carry the milk to the nipple, which is what a baby sucks when it's being breastfed. During puberty, as the breasts and nipples get bigger, the dark area around the nipple, called the aureola (pronounced or-ee-ola), also gets larger and goes a darker colour.

Most women's breasts differ slightly in shape and size from each other. The difference is often much more obvious while a girl is still growing. If she's really worried about looking lopsided, a slightly padded bra will help to even out the difference, but the chances are that no one else will notice. It shouldn't really matter in any case – we shouldn't have to feel pressured into living up to people's idea of what is or isn't 'perfect'.

Hairs sometimes grow around the nipples or in between the breasts. Shaving off these hairs only produces an uncomfortable stubble. Although it's really nothing to worry about, if it becomes very thick and dark and you don't like it, your doctor will tell you the best way to disguise or remove it.

Most girls think that their breasts are too big, too small, too

high or too droopy. The fashion pages in papers and magazines take a delight in telling us that breasts are supposed to
look small one season and large the next. It's certainly one
way of making us buy more clothes. The bra manufacturers
obviously try to sell as many bras as possible – there are
padded and wired bras for one fashion trend and 'no-bra' bras
for another. They can't have been too pleased when many
women decided to stop wearing them altogether. If a girl feels
better without a bra, then there's no point in wearing one. If
she finds that her breasts flop uncomfortably when she runs
or plays games, she may prefer to wear one. It's true that if
large breasts are unsupported they will eventually droop – but
who's to say that drooping breasts are any worse than those
that don't?

Magazines, Miss World contests and adverts are all geared
to make us think that every girl should have perfectly shaped
large breasts. (How often do you see a model with small
breasts on those advertisements for cigars, rum or pots of
paint?) Perhaps one day manufacturers will decide that their
products are good enough to sell on their own merit and don't
need big tits in order to make people spend their money. But
meanwhile this emphasis on the so-called 'perfect' large-
breasted female can make many girls with small breasts feel
inferior and somehow not very 'female'. And it can make girls
with large breasts feel worried that their bodies are little more
than toys for men to gawp at and play with.

Whether breasts are large or small makes no difference to
whether you'll be able to breastfeed your baby if and when
you want to. Nor does it make any difference to the amount of
pleasure and enjoyment you'll get from them. The breasts,
especially the nipples, of most girls (and some boys) are an
important part of enjoying sex. The size and shape make no
difference to the amount of sexual pleasure you get when
they're touched, stroked or kissed.

Vulva: The outer sex organs of a girl are called the vulva. This
consists of the mons pubis, outer lips, inner lips, clitoris,
urethra (pee-hole) and entrance to the vagina.

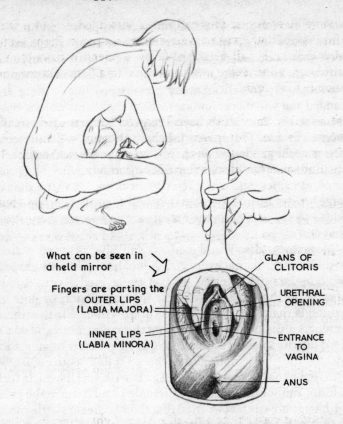

What can be seen in
a held mirror

GLANS OF
CLITORIS

Fingers are parting the
OUTER LIPS
(LABIA MAJORA)

URETHRAL
OPENING

INNER LIPS
(LABIA MINORA)

ENTRANCE
TO
VAGINA

ANUS

The best way for a girl to find out what her vagina looks like is to squat down and use a mirror to take a look.

There are many words used instead of the technical term – fanny, cunt, pussy are just some. In fact many girls don't use any word at all. And many more are brought up to think that they shouldn't touch or look at their sex organs. It's as if some people would have us believe that a girl's sex organs are dirty, unpleasant or simply don't exist. It doesn't sound strange to hear a boy talk about his penis as if it's a best friend called 'Willy' or 'John Thomas'. People tend to describe someone they don't think much of as a 'prick'. But when they *really* don't like someone they call her or him a 'cunt' – as if they think somehow a vagina is nastier than a penis. Perhaps one day girls will call their vulva by a friendly name too – although, admittedly, a 'Wilhelmina' or a 'Jane Thomasina' sounds a bit weird!

Mons pubis: Another technical term for the mons pubis is the Mons Veneris. This means 'Mount of Venus' – Venus being the ancient goddess of love. The mons pubis is the slightly raised mound on which the pubic hair grows.

Pubic hair: Also called pubes, bush. It grows on the mons pubis and on the outer lips. At first it is fine and colourless, and then it grows coarser and a much darker colour than the hair on the head.

Outer lips: The technical term is labia majora. Most of the time these lips lie close together to protect the more delicate skin and organs underneath.

Inner lips: The technical term is labia minora. When the outer lips are parted the darker, thinner and slightly slippery inner lips can be properly seen.

Clitoris: It consists of a head or glans (which means acorn) and a short stem or shaft. The glans is full of nerve endings which are what make the clitoris the most sensitive part of a girl's sex organs. It can usually be seen just poking out of a hood of skin at the top of the vulva where the inner lips meet. This hood of skin may have to be gently pushed back in order to see the clitoris properly. A girl who isn't sure where her clitoris is – and it's not always easy to find – should gently feel her vulva, and when she hits upon the most sensitive spot, it's pretty sure to be the clitoris. It can feel like a small sensitive bump about the size of a tiny pea.

The clitoris is made of spongy tissue with many small veins or blood vessels running through it. When a girl gets sexually excited a small ring of muscle at the base of the shaft tightens and stops the blood from flowing out. This makes the clitoris become firm and stiff and poke right out of its hood of skin. As sexual excitement dies down, the muscles relax, the blood flows in and out at the normal pace and the clitoris loses its stiffness and goes back in its hood. If all this sounds like what happens when a boy gets an erect penis – you're right. The clitoris and the penis both work in a very similar way. This is because during the very first stages of development in the womb, the tiny embryo (pronounced em-bree-o) of a girl is almost identical to that of a boy. And it's only as the embryo grows and starts developing that the cells growing into the sexual organs become the clitoris and vaginal lips in a girl, the penis and testicles in a boy.

Urethra (pronounced u-ree-thrah): This is the small opening just under the clitoris. It's also known as the pee-hole, because it's connected by a tube to the bladder, inside the body, which is where pee, or urine, collects. Pee comes out of the urethra.

Entrance to the vagina: The entrance or opening to the vagina is a ring of muscle which is usually small and tight. Slang words for the vagina include slit, crack, hole, twat. The muscles can relax, making the entrance wide enough to let a couple of fingers up into the vagina, a penis up into the vagina during sexual intercourse and to allow a baby to be born through it.

Hymen: Slang words include maidenhead and cherry. The entrance to the vagina may be partly or almost totally blocked by a thin layer of skin called the hymen. Some girls are born without a hymen or it may get broken at a young age quite naturally by riding a bike or horse or even by being constipated. A girl with a hymen may be able to see it in her mirror. If she can't push her fingers more than a few centimetres up into her vagina it means her hymen is still there. Some hymens have holes in them, but in any case it never completely seals off the vagina – the period will always be able to seep through.

What we look like – boys

Penis: There are many slang words for the penis: cock, tool, prick, dick, knob, willy, John Thomas, a man's best friend are some. Like the clitoris it's made up of two parts: the head is called the glans and the long part the shaft. The glans is the most sensitive part as it has thousands of nerve endings in it.

At the very tip of the head is the opening to a tube called the urethra which runs inside through the middle of the penis. Right inside the body this tube branches into two smaller tubes, with one going to the bladder and the other to the internal sex organs. The penis is made of spongy tissue with many small veins or blood vessels in it. When it's limp and little, blood flows in and out of the penis at a steady rate. When a boy gets sexually excited the ring of muscle inside the base of the shaft tightens and blood flows into the veins but not out. This makes his penis grow big and erect. As sexual excitement dies down, the muscles relax, the blood flows in and out at the normal rate and the penis goes back to being limp.

Foreskin: All boys are born with a thickish fold of skin which covers the glans. This is the foreskin and it's the equivalent to the hood of skin that protects the clitoris. The foreskin usually covers the head of the penis but it can be drawn back over the shaft. Under the foreskin a whitish waxy secretion called smegma – sometimes known as cock-cheese – is produced.

Circumcision is a minor operation which removes the foreskin. The most common difference between penises is whether or not this foreskin has been removed. Jewish boys are circumcised a few days after they're born; Moslem boys are circumcised when they're 8 or older. Baby boys may also

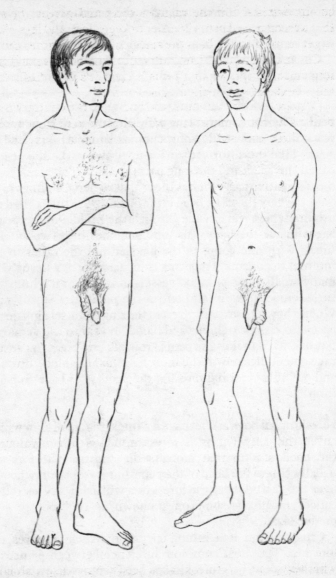

The boy on the left has a circumcised penis; the one on the right is uncircumcised.

be circumcised because many doctors and parents believe that a circumcised penis is easier to keep clean and less likely to get an infection, which the smegma can sometimes cause.

Circumcision makes no difference to a boy's sexual performance. In fact, when a penis is erect it's very difficult to tell whether it's been circumcised or not.

Despite all fears, rumours (and boasts) to the contrary most penises are the same size: usually about two or three inches when limp and about six inches when erect. But, like all

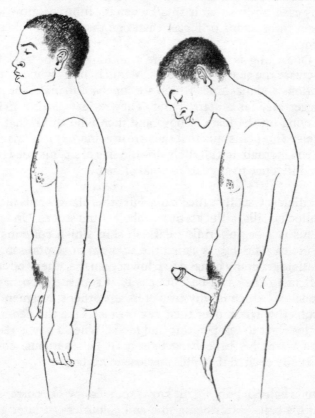

Although some boys may have quite a small penis when it is limp, most penises are roughly the same size and shape when they're erect.

averages, some are a bit smaller and others a bit larger. Boys (and men) can spend a lot of time worrying that their penis is too small or too thin, although there's really no need. The first thing to remember is that the penis is very sensitive to temperature and to how a boy feels. It may be that a boy who is convinced he has the smallest penis in the world has only been able to compare sizes at times when his fears are making his penis small, and the other boys around have been feeling warm and relaxed and so have a bigger-looking penis. And in any case, a penis that is small when it's limp can grow when erect to be as big or bigger than one that is large when it's limp.

One thing is certain: there's nothing anyone can do to increase the size of their penis. Manufacturers who advertise potions and machines which are supposed to make the penis bigger are, for a start, lying. They're just getting rich by playing on the fears of boys and men who think that girls prefer a big penis, and that they are in some way less 'manly' if theirs is small. It's all rubbish – the size of a penis need make no difference to anyone's sexual pleasure.

Testicles: Usually called balls, but other slang words include bollocks, pills, pillocks, nuts, cobblers and stones. Under the penis is a bag of crinkly darkish skin which contains two testicles. This bag is called the scrotum or scrotal sac. One testicle generally hangs down lower than the other – often the left one. They can be hurt easily if squeezed too hard or knocked (which is why cricketers and other sportsmen wear protective boxes over their sex organs). Like the penis, testicles react to temperature and mood. When a boy is relaxed and warm his balls hang loosely. If he's nervous, cold or sexually excited they pull up close to his body.

Pubic hair: Or pubes. This grows round a boy's sex organs and on his balls. After being fine and colourless, it later grows coarser and often a darker colour than the hair that grows on his head.

The inner sex organs

The hormones which change the shape and look of our bodies and outer sex organs also trigger off changes to our internal sex organs inside our bodies. Once our internal sex organs – or reproductive organs – are mature it means we are physically capable of having babies. When a girl reaches sexual maturity a ripe egg cell, called an ovum, is produced in her ovary. The first sign that this has happened is when she has her first period. When a boy reaches sexual maturity sperm is produced in his testicles. The first sign of this is when he has his first ejaculation of a fluid called semen (pronounced see-men), which contains millions of tiny sperm cells. The egg cell and the sperm cell are the two halves of human reproduction. Together the egg and sperm reproduce another human being – in other words, they make a baby.

REPRODUCTIVE ORGANS – GIRLS

Ovaries: Girls are born with two ovaries. They're made up of millions of tiny follicles, each with an unripe egg cell called an ovum inside. When a girl is physically mature, her ovaries are roughly the size and shape of an unshelled almond.

When she reaches puberty, her ovaries start to produce female sex hormones. These hormones do two things: they make the inner walls of her womb start to thicken with a rich lining of membrane and blood and they make an egg cell in one of her ovaries start to ripen. Very occasionally two egg cells are produced at the same time.

Under the influence of the hormones, a follicle with its ripening egg cells starts to move towards the surface of one or other ovary. When it's ripe, this follicle is released from its ovary. This is called ovulation. Some girls can tell when it's happening because they get a sudden sharp feeling of cramp in the lower part of their abdomen (stomach) on whichever side the follicle is being released.

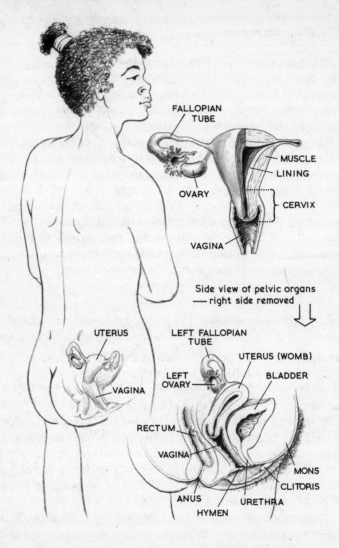

FALLOPIAN TUBE

MUSCLE

LINING

OVARY

CERVIX

VAGINA

Side view of pelvic organs
— right side removed

UTERUS

LEFT FALLOPIAN TUBE

UTERUS (WOMB)

BLADDER

LEFT OVARY

VAGINA

RECTUM

VAGINA

MONS

CLITORIS

ANUS

URETHRA

HYMEN

The uterus, or womb, from the back has its right side cut open to
show what it looks like inside. The fallopian tubes and ovaries –
like all our internal organs – naturally move around inside our
bodies, which is why no two pictures ever look exactly the same.

When the ripe egg pops off from its ovary, it is trapped in the end of the nearest fallopian tube.

Fallopian tubes: These two tubes are about three inches long. One end comes out of the top of the womb, the other end, which is fringed and funnel-shaped, wraps part way round an ovary. It is in the fallopian tubes that a baby will be conceived if a sperm cell meets and fertilizes an egg cell.

Separating from the follicle, the ripe egg is then trapped by the funnel-shaped fringed end of a fallopian tube. The ripe egg travels down the fallopian tube, taking about six and a half days to reach the womb.

Womb (or uterus): In a physically mature girl, the womb is about the size of a smallish clenched fist. It has thick walls of muscle that lie pressed against each other, rather like a balloon without any air in it. While the egg has been travelling down the fallopian tube, the walls of the womb have been developing a thick lining of membrane and blood. If the egg has been fertilized by a sperm, which means that the girl has become pregnant, it attaches itself to the lining and the growing baby is nourished and fed by this lining.

If the egg has not been fertilized by a sperm, meaning that the girl isn't pregnant, the egg has started to disintegrate by the time it reaches the womb. About twelve days after the egg reaches the womb, the muscles in the walls of the womb start to push out its thick lining through the cervix.

Cervix: This is the entrance to the womb. Running through the middle is a very thin passage. The lining of the womb is pushed through this passage into the vagina.

Vagina: The vagina is normally about three and a half inches long. It has walls of crinkled or ribbed membrane that normally lie flat against each other. It is a very flexible organ and can stretch to the size of more or less whatever is put in it, such as a finger or tampon, an erect penis or a baby when it is being born. (The vagina is also called the birth passage.)

The womb lining slips out of the vagina, past the hymen if there is one, and a girl has her period. It can take from two to eight days for the womb to push all the lining out.

PERIODS

The technical word for a period is menstruation. The membrane and blood from the womb is called menstrual blood or flow. The whole process from ovulation to having a period is known as the menstrual cycle. Menstruation comes from the Latin word *menses*, which means month – a misleading term because very few women have their periods on a regular monthly or 28-day basis.

Usually by the time a girl is fully sexually mature, her hormones produce another ripe egg in one or other of her ovaries several days after her period ends and the whole cycle starts all over again. But while her hormones are becoming adjusted, a girl often has to wait several months or perhaps more than a year before she has her next period. Eventually most women have their period every twenty-five to thirty-five days or so. But it's very rare for periods to happen absolutely regularly to the day each time. There are many reasons why a period can be early or late or missed altogether. Pregnancy is one reason, because during pregnancy hormones are produced in her body which prevent any more egg cells from ripening. Other reasons can be ill-health, emotional shock, fear of being pregnant or simply a change in climate or in normal routine.

Periods can last anything from two to eight days. Some girls have very light periods, others very heavy ones. The normal amount of blood lost is about five or six tablespoons – although because blood spreads and stains it can seem a lot more.

During the course of each period, whether it is heavy or light, girls need to wear something to absorb the blood and to protect their clothing. The next section discusses products that are readily available today from chemists and supermarkets.

SANITARY TOWEL OR TAMPON?

Either sanitary towels or tampons are used to absorb the period flow. There are many different brands to choose from. Sanitary towels are pads of absorbent cotton which fit under the entrance to the vagina inside pants or tights. Some have loops at each end to be attached to a belt which fastens round the waist. This sort tend to be rather big and lumpy – impossible to wear with tight trousers. But there are many different brands now which are small and compact and don't show at all, even in a bikini. It's worth shopping around for the type which feels most comfortable.

Many girls find tampons are more convenient. These are small finger-like wads of absorbent cotton wool that give internal protection. They are pushed up into the vagina where they expand to absorb the flow and fit comfortably in the vagina.

If a girl's hymen has not been broken, she may find it difficult to push the tampon in. But many hymens have holes in them which makes it possible to do this. If she does break her hymen when she pushes a tampon in, she may feel some pain. But it's often just a quick short sharp pain that quickly goes away and it's quite a good way of getting the whole business of hymen-breaking over and done with.

If putting a tampon in proves difficult it will be easier to wait until the period is over and then practise with a mirror to find out exactly where it should go. Another tip is to smear it with some sterile lubricating jelly, such as KY Jelly, that you can buy over the counter at a chemist's. This will help to slide it in more easily.

Pulling them out can sometimes cause problems. Each one has a small string attached to the end which hangs down outside the vagina. The best way to pull them out is to squat or stand with one leg raised on a chair or side of the bath, relax and give the string a gentle tug. If the string can't be found or the tampon seems to be stuck, it won't do any harm to wriggle a couple of fingers inside the vagina to find it and pull it out. If it's still stuck, don't panic. But don't leave it in either – it could cause an infection. If you can't ask a friend or

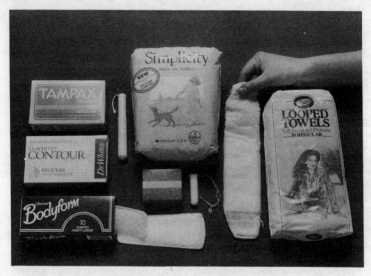

Sanitary towels, which go outside the vulva, and tampons, which go inside the vagina, come in many different shapes and sizes – find out which sort makes you feel most comfortable.

your mother to help you, go to your doctor and ask her or him to pull it out. This may sound like a drastic measure but doctors are often asked to do this.

Tampons come in different sizes – find one that feels most comfortable. One brand, called Tampax, has cardboard applicators to help put them in. The tampon is pushed out of its applicator into the vagina and you then throw the cardboard tube away.

Sanitary towels and tampons have to be changed regularly – several times a day is best and more often if the period is very heavy. Menstrual blood doesn't smell until it reaches the air when it can start to smell a bit unpleasant – so it's a good idea to change towels or tampons perhaps four or five times a day.

One of the best things about tampons is that they can be flushed down the toilet. Some sanitary towels are supposedly disposable in this way, but they often clog up the toilets.

Most towels have to be wrapped up and put in the dustbin or on the fire. Towels and tampons work out fairly expensive so some girls like to use small sponges with a little string attached. This can then be washed out and used again and again. Chemists sell all types of towels and tampons.

WHAT IT FEELS LIKE TO HAVE A PERIOD

Her first period can be a big event in a girl's life. It's proof that her body is maturing and that she'll be able to have babies if she wants to. But it can be a frightening experience, especially if no one has explained what is happening to her body.

Few people find it easy to talk openly about periods. Perhaps that's why so many slang words are used. It's often called being on the rag, on drip, feeling poorly, jam butties, aunty, monthlies, the time of the month, holy week, the curse and many other names. In the past there have been times when a woman who was having her period was thought to have magical powers. But more often than not she's been made to feel dirty, unclean or unlucky. Most unfairly, menstruating women have been accused of ruining crops, causing calves to be born dead and preventing the bread from rising. Small wonder it came to be called the curse!

There's still a lot of taboo surrounding the subject. Until very recently sanitary towels were rarely advertised and shops kept them well hidden from view. Many boys and men find the thought of periods so horrible that they won't have sex with someone who is having her period and are often too embarrassed to buy towels or tampons for her in the chemists. Girls who feel ill when they have their periods seldom like to say why they're feeling rotten.

There's no reason why someone who is having her period shouldn't have sex if she wants to – in fact it often helps relieve the pain of cramps to have orgasms and having a period is nothing to feel ashamed about. Perhaps if more people stopped to think why women have periods they wouldn't feel so shy or upset by the thought of them.

Having periods affects everyone in different ways. Some girls barely notice when they're having one. Others can feel grumpy, irritable or get a lot of pain. There are different sorts of pains that periods can cause. Some girls suffer from a constant dragging pain that can start several days before the period begins, called pre-menstrual tension, and some get sharper attacks of cramp-like pains actually during the period. Girls with irregular periods often suffer in particular from these pains (see also page 180). The pains often disappear as a girl gets older and her periods become more regular. What a girl needs if she's suffering from pains or if her period is making her feel low is not for everyone around her to feel embarrassed or repulsed, or even necessarily to ignore what's happening to her body, but to understand why she's feeling the way she is. There's no denying that periods can be a bit messy and sometimes inconvenient or painful. But they're a very natural part of being female.

There's a really good book which explains about periods in more detail. It's called *Have You Started Yet?* by Ruth Thomson (Piccolo, published by Pan).

REPRODUCTIVE ORGANS – BOYS

Testicles: Inside the scrotum or scrotal sac there are two glands called testes (pronounced test-ees) or testicles. Both of these are divided into several chambers which contain some very long, narrow, twisted tubes. When a boy reaches puberty the male sex hormone which is produced inside his testicles starts to cause sperm cells to be made inside these long narrow tubes. When the sperms have been made they pass out of each testicle into an epididymis (pronounced eppy-diddy-miss).

Epididymis: These organs lie on top of each testicle. They are made up of masses of larger tubes. Sperms are stored in each epididymis until a boy starts to get sexually excited and his penis grows erect. They are then pushed out of each epididymis by an automatic relaxing/contracting movement (a bit like swallowing) of the tubes into two seminal ducts.

Seminal ducts: These are two narrow tubes, technically known as the vas deferens, which go from each epididymis to a prostate gland. The sperms are pushed up the seminal ducts to this gland.

Prostate gland: This gland is inside the lower part of a boy's abdomen. It produces a fluid called seminal fluid. The sperms mix with this fluid and the mixture then passes out of the prostate gland into the seminal vesicles (pronounced vees-ickels).

Seminal vesicles: These are two small areas or sacs which store the sperm and seminal fluid mixture, which is called semen, until a boy reaches the peak of sexual excitement. At this point it leaves the vesicles and goes into a single tube called the urethra.

Urethra: This tube runs through the middle of the penis. The semen rushes through the urethra and comes out of the tip of the penis in four or five spurts. This is called ejaculation.

Inside a boy's body, at the point where the urethra joins the seminal vesicles, the urethra branches into two smaller tubes. One of these, as described above, goes to the inner sex organs. The other branch goes up to the bladder where pee collects. There is a tiny valve in the urethra tubes which means that when pee comes out of the bladder it bypasses the seminal vesicles, and carries on down through the penis and out of the hole in the tip. This valve makes sure that a boy can't pee and ejaculate at the same time.

When the penis is limp the valve opens the tube to the bladder. As soon as the penis starts to go erect, the valve closes the tube to the bladder and opens the tube to the sex organs.

Semen: Also called spunk, sex fluid, jism. Although there are about 300 million sperms in the average amount of semen ejaculated, they only form a very small portion of it. The bulk of it consists of the seminal fluid. The sperms are microscopic

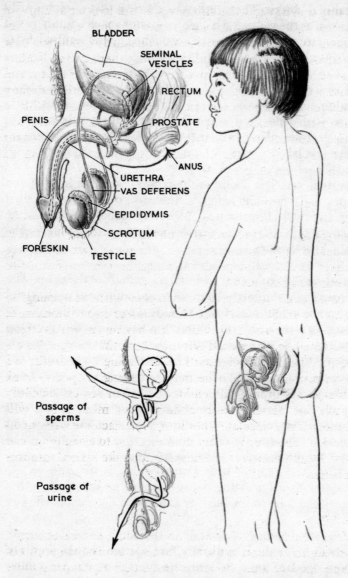

BLADDER

SEMINAL
VESICLES

RECTUM

PENIS

PROSTATE

ANUS

URETHRA

VAS DEFERENS

EPIDIDYMIS

SCROTUM

FORESKIN

TESTICLE

Passage of
sperms

Passage of
urine

**A boy's internal organs. A valve inside the urethra makes sure he
can't pee and ejaculate at the same time.**

– you couldn't tell the difference in the look or amount of semen if all 300 million were removed. Once a boy reaches sexual maturity, his testicles are constantly producing new sperms. There's no possibility of using them all up. If a boy has several ejaculations in a day, the amount of sperm and fluid will be slightly reduced – but there will still be many millions of sperm in each ejaculation for the rest of his life.

Semen is a milky, sticky, thickish liquid. It has a slightly salty, almost bitter taste. It's not poisonous. It can stain material if left – it soon hardens – but it's easy to wash off with soap and water.

EJACULATION

Also called shooting your load, or coming. Most boys start to ejaculate by the age of about 12. But some start earlier and others later. It all depends on when those hormones cause sperms to be produced.

Just as a girl's first period can happen without warning, so can a boy's first ejaculation. He may wake up one morning to discover semen on his pyjamas, not having known anything about it when it happened. (He may think that he's peed in his sleep.) When this happens it's called having a wet dream or a nocturnal emission. Or he may be feeling his penis, as he perhaps has throughout childhood, when semen suddenly spurts out. Having an erection doesn't mean a boy will automatically ejaculate – but it's rare to ejaculate without an erection. The time it takes from erection to ejaculation can vary. It can take a few seconds or it can take several minutes or longer.

ERECTIONS

Also called having a hard on, on the bonk, or feeling horny. Getting an erection is usually, but not always, the result of some kind of sexy or erotic influence. It happens quite naturally, a bit like blushing. Many boys after the age of 11 or so find that they get erections for no obvious reason at all and sometimes many a day. It can happen in the gym, on the top of a bus, at the breakfast table – and by just wondering when it will happen. This is quite natural, and sudden, unexpected and often unwanted erections stop happening after a time. But it can be embarrassing. An erection isn't always the easiest thing in the world to hide. The best thing to do is to try thinking about something else entirely. Concentrating on your kid brother or your homework can do wonders to make your penis shrink. Having an erection is a perfectly normal thing, but you might get a bit of a pain or ache in your balls and the lower part of your stomach after a while. Having an ejaculation often helps to ease this pain.

WET DREAMS

Both girls and boys have wet dreams (or dreams in which they reach a peak of sexual excitement) but girls don't ejaculate. The sort of dream that makes a boy ejaculate is often very sexy. It's quite natural to dream about having sex with someone you know well of the same or opposite sex even though in the daytime you mightn't think about them in a sexy way at all. Or you may dream about someone of either sex whom you fancy. The dreams may involve violent situations. No one has yet found a way of controlling our dreams and hopefully they never will. And however violent or odd a dream may be, having it doesn't mean that you're automatically going to grow up to be a rapist or to be hopelessly in love with your brother or mother!

Many boys hate waking up to find semen all over their pyjamas and sheets. If you want to avoid this, try sleeping in underpants which can then be washed out the next morning, or give yourself an ejaculation before you go to sleep, and use a paper handkerchief to absorb the semen.

The good thing about having a wet dream and ejaculating is that it's a sure sign of reaching sexual maturity, just as periods are for a girl. But not every boy has them. He may only ejaculate when he masturbates or he may never ejaculate until he has sex. Most men ejaculate at some time in their lives, but if they don't, the sperms just disintegrate, and are absorbed into the body without causing any harm.

Egg and sperm together: fertilization

A girl can only get pregnant if a ripe egg cell in her fallopian tubes is fertilized by a sperm cell.

When a couple have sexual intercourse the man puts his erect penis into a woman's vagina. When he ejaculates the millions of sperms in his semen swim blindly around in the vagina, up through the small passage in the entrance to the womb (cervix) and into the womb (uterus).

From the womb, sperms swim into the fallopian tubes. If there's a ripe egg cell in one of the fallopian tubes, a sperm may enter and fertilize it. It's at this point that a baby is conceived. If, as occasionally happens, a fertilized egg splits into two, identical twins will be produced. Sometimes two ripe egg cells develop at the same time; if they are both fertilized, non-identical twins will be the result.

Another way in which women can get pregnant is by having some sperms inserted into their womb scientifically by a doctor. It's been discovered that sperms can be kept alive and unharmed for several years by freezing them. The sperms can then be used by women who haven't been able to get pregnant by a man who is infertile (which means that his body doesn't produce sperms). Lesbian women, women who don't want to have sex with a man because they feel sexually attracted to women rather than men, can also have babies in this way. Several sperm banks have been set up for these purposes, and it's called having a child by A.I.D. which stands for Artificial Insemination by Donor, meaning the artificial sowing of the sperm seed. Because the semen which contains the sperm can carry the virus which causes the illness AIDS (not to be confused with A.I.D. without the S at the end), some women are wary of getting pregnant in this way. But all sperm in these banks are now tested for AIDS and every man (or donor) who offers his sperm is also tested to check that he doesn't have the virus.

CHAPTER THREE

Who Am I?

What's normal?

The sex organs of all girls look more or less the same. So do the sex organs of boys. But obviously, just as no two people develop at exactly the same pace or in the same way, no two people are ever exactly alike either. But the society we live in tries to make us feel as if we should all be the same: women like all other women and men like all other men. People tend to judge each other by what society as a whole seems to think of as 'normal'. And being normal is often assumed to be whatever those who control society do and think. This is highly unfair on those who don't fit into the patterns laid down. Treating differently those who don't fit into the norm is called discrimination. Treating them badly is called being intolerant.

Femininity and masculinity

In our society girls are brought up to be soft, gentle and passive. And boys are brought up to be tough and aggressive. This isn't always done deliberately. But think of the difference between the sort of comics and books that are written for girls and boys. Most often you find that girls get to read about gentle things, while boys' books are about war and fighting. It used to be thought that only men should go out to work, and that this was 'manly', and that women should stay behind at home because it was 'womanly' to cook and look after babies and do the housework. Unemployment has changed this picture quite a bit. So has feminism. Many

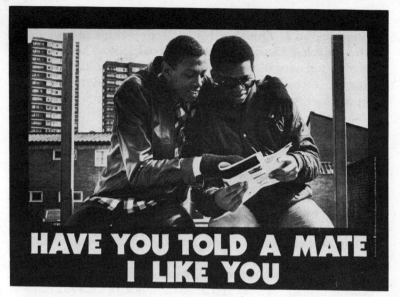

HAVE YOU TOLD A MATE
I LIKE YOU

Many boys feel they have to be so tough and macho that they never know how good it feels to express their feelings.

people have learned that women can be just as womanly if they go out to work and that men were missing out on some of the softer, more lovely parts of life if they ignored every-thing that women had traditionally always done.

But it hasn't changed totally. Many still think it's some-how unfeminine for a girl to ask a boy out for a date or to admit that she gets turned on sexually. And it's thought to be 'unmasculine' for a boy to enjoy cooking or let his girlfriend buy him a drink. Treating girls and boys differently like this is called having double standards. Expecting everyone to be-have in a certain way just because of their sex when maybe they don't feel like fitting into the so-called 'normal' way of acting causes a lot of unhappiness.

A boy, for example, is often almost expected to sleep around a bit with as many girls as he can while he's young. Girls, on the other hand, are expected to save themselves and remain virgins until they marry. The words 'slut' or 'slag' are often used to describe a girl who sleeps around, or even one who only has had more than one boyfriend. These words aren't often used to describe a boy who does the same thing. Boys are often allowed to stay out late. Girls find that they're expected to stay at home – often to babysit – or be in earlier than boys.

Making everyone fit into a neatly labelled box like this is unfair on those who don't fit the generally accepted view. Girls who want to be themselves and who enjoy playing football or who want to be engineers are often thought to be slightly odd or 'masculine'. Boys who cry when they're sad – a perfectly normal thing for all human beings – or who want to be nurses are accused of being 'sissy'. Do we really want to live in a society where we can't choose who we want to be?

It's widely believed that girls are not only physically weaker than boys but also more weak-minded. A girl is just as capable of learning how to change the wheel of a car as a boy – but you don't see many girls in mechanics lessons. And lots of men think they have to come to the aid of women (stupidly sometimes called 'the weaker sex') like knights on their chargers. Some years ago in Israel, Members of Parliament were discussing the problem of the large number of women who were attacked in the streets at night. To protect the women, the mainly male MPs kindly suggested passing a law to make all women be in their homes by ten o'clock. But the Prime Minister (a woman) pointed out that as it was the men who were doing the attacking, it was they who should be banned from the streets, not the women!

Heterosexuality, homosexuality, bisexuality

Society's mania for labelling people and making those who don't fit in feel different and odd also applies to how some people think about sexuality. It's assumed to be automatic and normal for women and men to be attracted to members of the opposite sex. This is true for the majority of people –

that's to say, most people are heterosexual. (*Hetero* is a Greek word meaning 'other'.) But it isn't true for everyone. Quite a lot of people, probably about one in ten, are attracted to members of the same sex. The technical word for them is homosexual, from the Greek word *homos*, meaning 'same'. (Not to be confused with a similar word, *homo*, meaning 'humankind'.) Bisexuals are people who are attracted sexually to both sexes. Those who aren't attracted by anyone are called asexual. But just because they're not a majority doesn't mean they're not normal or that their sex lives are 'unnatural'. It feels perfectly normal to them.

There have been lots of theories why some of us are heterosexual while others are homosexual or bisexual, but none of them have ever been very satisfactory. The chemical make-up of our bodies may have something to do with it. But there are no hard and fast rules. It's no good thinking that because someone had a very powerful mother and a weak father that they'll automatically turn out to be homosexual. This may happen and it may not.

In the past there have been some societies in which it was perfectly OK for people to be homosexual or bisexual. But in the Western world today, being anything other than heterosexual is not easy. Even though homosexuality doesn't harm anyone, homosexuals are often discriminated against and treated with a lot of intolerance. Perhaps many heterosexuals are scared that there's a bit of homosexuality in themselves. Or maybe their intolerance comes from a very common fear of anyone who is different.

Female homosexuals call themselves lesbians – the word comes from Lesbos, a Greek island where a very fine poet called Sappho wrote poems about the love between women in ancient times. Many male homosexuals call themselves gays – not because they're always bright and lively, but because they're happy to have discovered this about themselves and know it's nothing to be ashamed of. When lesbians and gays admit to themselves and to the rest of the world that they are homosexual, it's called 'coming out'. But intolerant non-gays (sometimes called straights) go on calling them cruel and insulting names such as queers, pooves, poufters, pansies, fairies, queens, faggots and dykes. Not only are gays called hurtful names, but they are also treated in many hurtful ways.

How we enjoy sex should be a matter for ourselves to choose. There's every reason to believe that if any one of us found ourselves stranded on a desert island with only one person of the same sex for company, we'd find it both easy and natural to have a homosexual relationship. This is presumably why many prisoners, soldiers and others who find themselves without members of the opposite sex around enjoy homosexual relationships. Many people, if left to their own natural instincts, would probably discover that they were bisexual and could enjoy sexual relationships with both women and men. But society, with its passion for trying to make us all the same, tries to make us hold back these instincts. Holding back a natural sexual instinct can make people feel bewildered and unhappy.

Neither heterosexuality nor homosexuality is some sort of dangerous drug that you get hooked on for the rest of your life. A very large number of women and men who would not think of themselves as lesbian or gay have had some kind of homosexual experience at some time in their lives. Some girls and boys experiment with a partner of their own sex before they get to a relationship with someone of the opposite sex. Certainly around puberty many of us go through a time when we don't have a lot of time for the opposite sex and have strong sexual feelings for people of the same sex. If we have homosexual experiences it isn't going to harm us any more than if we have sexual experiences with the opposite sex and in the end find out that we prefer to be lesbian or gay. The point is to realize that we all have different tastes, and to be in a minority doesn't make anyone 'abnormal' or wrong.

Being lesbian or gay

As about one in ten people is lesbian or gay, that means there are probably around six million lesbians and gays in the

UK. According to the way society likes to put everyone into neatly defined and clearly labelled boxes, gays are supposed to have limp wrists, talk with lisps, have rounded hips and act like women – however it is that women are supposed to act. And lesbians are supposed to be tough types with gruff voices, short-back-and-sides hairstyles, and to dress and act like men. How wrong can you get! Of course some lesbians and gays do live up to this picture – just as some straight women and men conform to an image of what many people think it means to look like a woman or a man. But the way people look or dress doesn't have to have anything to do with how they enjoy sex.

Business women and men, factory-workers, pop stars, politicians, teachers – there's no group of people that doesn't have its proportion of lesbians and gays. But perhaps because some groups of people tend to be more tolerant of others, many lesbians and homosexuals have doubtless been attracted to the sort of jobs where they will find fellow workers who will treat them with respect as fellow human beings and not as outcasts.

Sexually, lesbians and gays have the same sort of relationships as heterosexuals. They may have sex for fun, out of curiosity, for friendship, or because they're in love. One image of gays is that they are very promiscuous, tending to have lots of different partners and not settling down with one person. There are many, many gays who do have steady single relationships. And there are many, many straights who sleep around and who are unfaithful to their partners. When they're busy attacking gays, intolerant people tend to forget the number of married men who go to prostitutes for sex.

However, it is probably true that gays – more than lesbians – have tended to have more sexual relationships than many straights. This may be partly because in a society that makes it difficult for homosexuals to come out and admit that they're gay, even though it is perfectly legal, they find it difficult to sort out their own feelings. It's probably also true that once a gay has come out, he finds it liberating to have a lot of different partners.

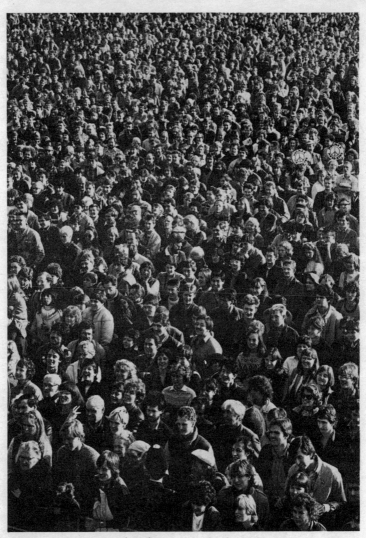

About one in ten people is homosexual. There's no way you can tell if people are lesbian or gay just by looking at them.

When the AIDS illness arrived, some people – those who were anti-gay – tried to make us believe that the reason why mostly gays had the disease was because they were promiscuous. This is now known to be absurd, although this hasn't stopped a lot of people from still thinking it. Yes, statistically speaking the more partners you have, the more likely you are to meet someone who has the infection. But it isn't simply having lots of different partners in itself that gives anyone AIDS. Just one sexual encounter with someone who is infected can give you the virus that can lead to AIDS. And in any case, it isn't only gays who can get AIDS – it's now known that everyone is at risk, straights and gays. For more information about AIDS and how to avoid it see pages 160–67.

A lot of people are very curious about what lesbians and gays do in bed. The answer is: much the same as straights. They give and get sexual pleasure by kissing, cuddling, feeling and stimulating their partner's genitals with their hands and their mouths. For lesbians and gays, sex is as natural as it is for anyone else. What they do and how they give and get love and sexual pleasure is up to them as individuals. Because AIDS first hit mostly the gay community in the Western world, gays more than any other group of people now practise safer sex. This means not coming into contact with any of the fluids in the body which carry the virus. Straights are taking a bit longer to realize that caring for someone sexually now means practising safer sex.

In the past, gays have been treated very inhumanely. Until 1967 male homosexuality was actually illegal in Great Britain – it still is in the Isle of Man, Jersey and the Republic of Ireland. Lesbianism has never been illegal, although it's never been easy for lesbians to admit their love for each other openly. For a long time even a novel which referred to female or male homosexuality was likely to be banned. It is still impossible for lesbians and gays to marry and only very recently have lesbians been allowed to adopt children. Gays still have to fight for this right. Due to some very confused thinking, some people believe that gays should not be allowed to look after children. They think they might harm them in some way. In fact, most children who are abused sexually (and this is presumably what these people are really worried about) are girls who are abused by heterosexual men. Of course, some young boys are sexually abused by gay paedophiles (adults who are sexually attracted to children). But it makes no more sense to think that all gays are paedophiles than it does to think that all straight men want to harm young girls.

Even though male homosexuality is not illegal, the law continues to discriminate against homosexuals and to treat them differently from heterosexuals. These are some of the differences:

—The age of consent for gays is 21; for everyone else it is 16 (in the Republic of Ireland, 17).
—Gays are only allowed to enjoy sex 'in private'. This means that no one else can even be in the same house, flat or hotel, even if they don't mind at all. There is no such law for straights, who are perfectly free to enjoy sex in any house or hotel.
—Gays under 21 who have sex (even if they're 20 years and 11 months old) are breaking the law. Girls under 16 who have sex are not.
—Homosexuality is still illegal for members of the armed services and the Merchant Navy.

On the whole, lesbians and gays are finding it easier to be open about their sexual preference than they used to be. AIDS, however, has been seized upon as an excuse for some intolerant people to make it more difficult than it once was. Some politicians who would certainly never physically beat up a gay find it acceptable to attack them verbally. The psychological damage this can cause can be just as harmful as a punch in the face. And teaching others to be intolerant causes damage to society as well. Thinking anyone is sinful or that they should be treated badly simply because they're different is no way for a civilized society to progress. It's what Hitler thought when, during the Second World War, he murdered millions of Jews, gipsies, the disabled, homosexuals and trade unionists in extermination camps because he considered them inferior beings – not people at all.

But because of a general atmosphere of intolerance, many lesbians and gays find life very difficult. Some get to feel so hung up about their homosexuality that they marry non-gays in the hope that this will somehow 'cure' them. They usually end up in a position of being hurt, even more scared, and hurting the person they married. Homosexuality isn't an illness – it's simply a matter of a sexual instinct that is directed towards someone of the same sex.

Transvestites and transsexuals

Some people think that lesbians really want to be men and that gays really want to be women. This isn't so. People who like dressing up in the clothes of the opposite sex are called transvestites. Transvestites can be either straight or gay. Some want to cross-dress in order to get sexually aroused; many do it simply because it makes them feel more like 'themselves'. The law usually ignores women transvestites and male entertainers who perform drag acts. But men who like to wear women's clothes and make-up can find themselves in trouble with the law for 'insulting behaviour' or 'causing a breach of the peace', which both carry prison sentences of up to six months. Quite why it is that a woman who wears a shirt and jeans is not thought to be insulting, while a man who likes dresses is insulting, is beyond understanding. But that's what the law says, and as long as it stays like that male transvestites shouldn't risk dressing up in public places.

People who do want to change their sex are called transsexuals. Identifying with the opposite sex usually takes place at a very early age; it often has something to do with a hormonal imbalance that they're born with, although not necessarily. They grow up feeling trapped inside a body of the wrong sex. To change sex totally, hormone treatment, several operations and therapy with a sex counsellor are necessary. By law, no doctor can give any of this treatment until a person is 18.

Want some help?

Discovering that you are or might be a lesbian or gay, or that you may be a transvestite or transsexual, can come as something of a shock. Society, after all, has been impressing on you that to be different is to be 'abnormal'. If you think that you might want legal help, moral support or advice, contact one of the organizations mentioned on page 199. And, if you're just not sure quite what your problem is, don't worry that any of these organizations will try to convert you. They're not into getting new recruits, they're there in order to help solve your problem, whether it's big or little.

For a really good book which explains more about being straight, gay, lesbian or bisexual, read *So You Think You're Attracted to the Same Sex?* by John Hart (Penguin).

CHAPTER FOUR

Masturbation

There are countless words for masturbating: wanking, fiddling, playing with yourself, jacking off, jerking off, tossing off, bringing yourself off are just some of them.

Very simply, masturbating means rubbing your clitoris or penis – usually, though not always, with your hand – in order to get sexually excited and often (though again not always) give yourself an orgasm. It gives you a good feeling and it's a way of getting to know how your body works and responds to sexual excitement.

A girl gets sexually excited by feeling her genitals, especially her clitoris. As she reaches the peak of excitement her whole body feels in tune with the feelings in her sex organs. Very often her vagina, and maybe her pee-hole (urethra), produces a fluid which makes her external organs (vulva) wet. When she reaches the peak or climax of pleasure, the muscles in her vagina start to move in spasms and the feelings of tenseness and excitement mingle with a feeling of release and satisfaction. This all sounds very dramatic – and it can be, but it can also be like a soft, warm, gentle sigh of pleasure.

A boy gets much the same sensations from rubbing his penis. The movement gives him an erection and he reaches a peak of sexual excitement. This feeling spreads from his sex organs to the whole of his body. At the climax, semen comes out of the hole in the tip of his penis, in four or five spurts. The feeling of tenseness and excitement mixes into a feeling of release and satisfaction. His penis goes limp almost immediately afterwards and his body goes back to being relaxed.

Expressions for having an orgasm, such as coming, arriving

or getting there, are quite good descriptions for what it can feel like.

The myths

Doctors have known for years that masturbating is totally harmless, but many people still have the suspicion lurking in the back of their minds that it's a dangerous, harmful or even wicked thing to do. Many of the jokes and limericks about wanking reflect this suspicion:

> There was a young man named Hank
> Who often enjoyed a good wank
> But he once gave a cough
> And his penis dropped off
> To be frank, Hank regrets learning to wank.

Most of us have heard at some time or other that masturbating can:

—make you blind
—drive you mad
—make you sterile and unable to have babies
—ruin a marriage
—dry up the brain
—alter the shape of your sex organs
—drain the 'vital juices'
—give you spots
—give you cancer
—give you stomach aches
—give you headaches
—put hairs on your palms

But NONE of these things is true. There's absolutely NO evidence of any kind at all of a connection between masturbating and madness or any illness.

THERE WAS A YOUNG LADY NAMED . . .

There's another myth about masturbating which suggests that it's not something girls do. It is true that many more boys do it than girls but the reason for this is not because girls don't have sexual feelings but because of the difference in their bodies and the different ways in which they're brought up sexually. Many boys, even in this day and age, are discouraged from masturbating, but parents can't tell their sons not to touch their penis or they wouldn't be able to pee. But parents often firmly discourage their daughters from playing with their sex organs. Some girls are told outright lies, like their sex organs will drop off if they touch themselves. This means that girls, even more than boys, grow up thinking that to feel themselves is somehow 'naughty' or 'wrong' or in some way dangerous. Of course some girls go right ahead and learn how to masturbate, and others teach themselves when they're much older. But some don't, and many tend to feel very guilty about getting good sexual feelings from masturbating. And this feeling of guilt can spread to their whole attitude towards all sex.

Women and girls of all ages enjoy masturbating every bit as much as men and boys. Masturbating can't harm anyone, so no one should feel guilty or scared about it.

SO WHY ALL THE MYTHS?

In the past the most dreadful punishments were handed out to girls and boys found masturbating. Up to the nineteenth century they might have had their arms bound to their sides in splints, their thighs blistered with hot irons, some boys were circumcised (although this never stopped any boy from wanking) and some girls had their clitoris removed. Some unfortunate men in mental hospitals who were often thought by the authorities to masturbate 'too much' had their penis chopped off altogether.

The main reason for all this was that many people were convinced that sex was wrong unless it took place between a married couple who wanted to have a baby. This was certainly the opinion of most religious people, who could find passages from the Bible to support their view. It's easy to see why masturbation, which obviously can't get anyone pregnant, came to be thought of as sinful and unnatural.

Attitudes like this die hard. For some religious and more traditionally-minded people the feeling that masturbating is wrong or immoral lives on. Your parents, teachers or doctors may have been brought up along these lines and may still think like this.

If your own moral sense or religious beliefs tell you that sex *is* only for having babies or you want to conform to your parents' point of view, and they think it's wrong, then masturbating may not be for you. There's no sense in doing anything that you strongly believe to be wrong. But if you do masturbate and enjoy the feelings you get, don't worry that it will make you ill or damage you in any way. It won't.

How girls masturbate

There isn't any one, or a right or wrong, way in which to masturbate. There are so many different ways that it's impossible to mention them all but the majority of girls use a finger, several fingers or their whole hand to rub gently and rhythmically over the clitoris until they reach orgasm. Or they may use a firmer action over the whole vaginal area, perhaps using both hands for greater pressure. The action usually gets faster and faster until they come.

Rubbing against a dry clitoris can sometimes make it feel a bit sore, so use some of the wetness produced inside the vagina, some spit or something gentle like KY Jelly that you can buy from the chemist.

A few find that they can bring themselves off by using the muscles in their vagina. This usually needs a bit of practice – if you don't know where these muscles are or how to make them contract you can try the following exercise: when you're peeing, tighten the muscles in your vaginal area to hold back the pee for a little while. When you've found out where these muscles are you can practise making them contract and relax any time during the day – no one will notice what you're doing.

Another way of masturbating is to use a sheet, pillow or flannel and pull it back and forwards over the clitoris. Some like to put a finger or two in their vagina or anus because at the peak of an orgasm the muscles in both these organs contract in spasms. Spraying the clitoris and vagina with a jet of water can also give an orgasm. Some girls have learned how to come in this way because they were told never to touch themselves and so always washed their vaginas under the tap or used a shower spray. You may find you have an orgasm by touching your nipples, or your clitoris and a nipple at the same time, or by crossing your legs and rubbing them together.

Some women masturbate with sex toys. Vibrators and dildoes (sometimes called dildols) are penis-shaped objects made of rubber or plastic. Vibrators are powered by batteries or can be plugged into the electricity to make them shake or vibrate slightly. They are used to play gently over the clitoris and sex organs or put inside the vagina – although penetration is certainly not the only way women enjoy sex. These sex toys often cost a lot of money and there are many much cheaper things around the house which do just as well. Obviously nothing should be used that might irritate or harm the tender skin of the sex organs. But no one should feel guilty because they like to use something other than their fingers. Sex toys should be thoroughly washed after you've used them. And because it's just about possible for the virus that can lead to AIDS to be carried by a sex toy, never lend them to anyone else.

How long it takes to masturbate can vary. Much depends on how long it takes to get in the right mood – this can take a minute or two or it can take up to an hour or more. Many girls find that it takes them a long time to learn how to masturbate and reach an orgasm. But whether or not they come, most girls find it enjoyable and exciting.

How boys masturbate

One way is to make a fist, hold the penis quite firmly in it and jerk the hand up and down with a shaking action that gets faster and faster as the excitement builds up. A boy who hasn't been circumcised like to bring the foreskin up and down over the head of the penis. Some boys prefer a less vigorous method and they stroke the head of the penis with their finger tips. Or they may masturbate without using their hands at all by lying on their stomachs and pushing their bodies up and down to make their penis rub against the bed or ground.

Some boys find that it increases their pleasure to push a finger up their anus. It's a very bad idea to push anything inside the penis because of the danger of harming the delicate tissue inside or of getting an infection.

Some boys like to put the inner cardboard tube from a toilet-paper roll on their penis. Or they use butter, oil or soapy water to make the penis feel nice and slippery. There's probably nothing that hasn't been used by someone at some time or other. It occurs to most boys to try to suck their penis – although most find this best left to india-rubber men!

Can masturbating do any good?

It can certainly relieve tension. Many sports people are discouraged from masturbating before a game or a race. This is probably all part of the old-fashioned view that masturbating is bad for you and weakens your body by draining it of its 'vital juices' (whatever they might be). Some athletes say they've given their best record-breaking performances after they've had an orgasm. It all depends on whether you're the sort of person who needs to be tense before a performance or prefers to feel relaxed. The amount of energy you use up when you masturbate is probably about the same as walking up a flight of stairs – and no athlete has ever been told to stay at ground level before a race.

Another thing in favour of masturbating is that it helps you to get to know your own body. It needn't be just a mechanical means of relieving tension, like peeing is a mechanical means of emptying your bladder. It's a way of enjoying sex on your own if you can't or don't want to have sex with someone else.

Masturbating can also take your mind off any problems you may have. This is why some people with worries and problems masturbate a lot. You can't masturbate 'too much', but wanking doesn't solve your problems. And if you spend most of your time doing nothing but masturbating and thinking about it you'll never get round to finding any solutions.

Masturbating is usually a very private thing, although some girls and boys experiment by doing it in groups. But it's also something that couples often enjoy doing. It's an important part of safer sex because it means that no body fluids such as semen, vaginal fluid or period blood, which in an infected person carry the virus that causes AIDS, can enter their partner's body. Obviously if the boy masturbates over a part of his partner's body which has a scratch or cut then his semen will enter the other's body directly. Many couples who practise safer sex use a condom whether they're having sexual intercourse or masturbating. And covering any sores or scratches with a waterproof plaster is also a good idea.

If you are masturbating in private, the big fear can be that you'll be discovered by your parents or by someone who walks into your room without knocking and waiting first. If this does happen to you, and whoever it is looks horrified, try to figure out why they're horrified. It could well be that they disapprove altogether (even though the chances are that they used to masturbate themselves and probably still do), in which case you'll have to find a more private place in future. Or it could be simply that *they're* upset that *you* might be upset to be found doing something that you wanted to do in private.

Enjoying a good wank can be very pleasurable – many women say that the orgasm they get from masturbating is more intense than when they reach orgasm through sexual intercourse. Some people masturbate because they're frightened of having a relationship with someone else. But no one should worry that just because they masturbate they'll never fully enjoy sex with a partner. Every single sexual experience whether with a partner or on your own is different each and every time. Ignore the myth that suggests that if you masturbate and enjoy it you'll never be able to have a good sexual relationship with another person – this simply isn't true.

Some people think of masturbation as a poor substitute for having sex with someone else. Perhaps that's why someone who mucks around and never gets down to the real thing in life is often called 'a wanker'. But wanking and coming can make people feel very good. And it is a way of getting sexual pleasure and satisfaction and learning how to love your body.

Finally: You don't *have* to masturbate if you don't want to. Some girls and boys never feel the need. This doesn't mean that you're never going to enjoy sex. Different people have different needs at various times and ages. No one should feel that they must have sex just because they think everyone else is having it. Only you will be able to tell whether you want it, and when and how you want it.

CHAPTER FIVE

Orgasms

Slang words for having an orgasm and the peak or climax of an orgasm are mostly connected with travelling – they include coming or having a come, getting there, arriving and making it. You can have an orgasm either by masturbating or by having sex with someone else.

Having an orgasm follows a similar physical pattern for both girls and boys, although the feelings and sensation often differ, both from time to time and from person to person. First of all we get aroused and our bodies start to feel ready for sex. Sexual excitement builds up to a high level, and, at the peak, the sex organs contract in a series of spasms and a feeling of release and sexual pleasure flows through the whole body.

Most boys know what it's like to have an orgasm before they ever have sex with anyone because masturbating and ejaculating are a normal part of their lives. It's obvious when a boy comes – semen spurts out of the end of his penis. Ejaculation during orgasm only happens once puberty has arrived; before puberty, orgasm is the pleasurable feeling without the ejaculation of seminal fluid. A girl doesn't have such an obvious physical sign and it's less easy to tell when she comes. Writers who have tried to describe the female orgasm tend to go in for some very lurid and flowery writing – waves crashing overhead, thunder and lightning booming and flashing around and the occasional earthquake!

It's very easy to be misled by such over-dramatic descriptions. Some girls can be waiting so intently for the flashes and booms that they either don't have an orgasm or don't realize they've had one when they have. The truth is that all women respond differently and each orgasm can vary in intensity. Sometimes an orgasm can slip out like a quiet happy sigh. At other times it can be a very powerful feeling that shakes the whole body and totally invades the mind.

For many girls, having an orgasm is something they have to learn by masturbating. If a girl can find out for herself how her body responds and likes to be stimulated, it'll be easier for her to enjoy sex to the full with someone else if and when she wants to because she'll be able to show her sex partner how her particular body works.

Getting turned on

Our bodies need to be turned on (or sexually stimulated and aroused as it's called) in order to start to feel ready for sex. You can get aroused in lots of ways, and direct contact with the penis or clitoris isn't the only way to get excited. Kissing, cuddling, touching, stroking, caressing your own or another's body in any number of places – lips, breasts, back, legs, head, hair or anywhere that feels good – can start to turn you on. Or you may feel aroused by seeing someone you fancy, by looking at sexy books, magazines or films or just having sexy thoughts.

Many people enjoy thinking or fantasizing about sex while they masturbate or have sex with someone. It often helps get you into a sexy mood and reach an orgasm more easily. What you think about when you masturbate can range from imagining or remembering being kissed to having sexual intercourse. To some extent our fantasies come from the kind of world we live in. It's quite natural to fantasize about having sex with someone you know well (a friend, someone in your family, a teacher), with someone of the same or opposite sex, about going with or being a prostitute or about raping someone or being raped. There's no limit to what people can fantasize about and there's no need to be scared about even quite violent fantasies. You might day-dream – or fantasize – about being a pop star or winning an Olympic Gold Medal, but as long as you don't act like a super-star or expect to be treated as one, then no one is going to think you odd. The same thing applies to sexual fantasies. As long as you don't think you have to act out your wilder sex thoughts, there's nothing to worry about.

Being sexually aroused is a good feeling, no matter who or what turns you on. Some people would like to ban all sexy books and films – perhaps because deep down what they're really complaining about is that people enjoy getting sexual feelings. But it's possible to be turned on by listening to classical music or by riding on a bus. No one has yet suggested that Beethoven or public transport should be banned.

Having an orgasm – girls

It used to be thought that the vagina was the centre of a girl's orgasm and that the only way for her to come was to have something in her vagina moving up and down. This helped to make some men – and women – think that unless there was a man around with an erect penis women couldn't enjoy sex. But then it was noticed that most women needed to have their clitoris stimulated in order to come. This led to another myth: that women could have two sorts of orgasms, one in the clitoris and one in the vagina. In fact there is only one kind of orgasm and it involves all the sex organs.

Orgasms feel different for different people and at different times, but there are certain physical changes that happen to their bodies when they come. As a girl gets sexually aroused and excited her nipples become firm and erect and her breasts swell slightly. In some girls this shows a lot, in others it's barely noticeable. The feelings are passed to her sex organs. The clitoris becomes firm and pokes out of its hood of skin which makes it easier to stimulate. Blood rushes to the sex organs, which go a darker pinky-red colour in much the same way as your face goes red when you blush. The outer lips become firmer and separate from each other. Some girls find that the whole of the front of their bodies, including their faces, become warm and flushed.

The vagina reacts to excitement in several ways. The

innermost two thirds stretches and the walls of the outer third, just inside the entrance, swell out and secrete a clear or slightly whitish fluid that can leak out and make the whole of the outer sex organs wet. All the muscles in her body tense up and breathing gets faster. Just before the peak or climax the clitoris, still firm, goes back into its hood.

The climax of an orgasm involves a series of short rhythmical spasms in the walls of the outer, third, part of the vagina. These spasms spread up to the womb, to all the sex organs and sometimes to the whole body. The muscles of the anus also usually contract in spasms, which is why some people like to put a finger in their anus to add to their pleasure.

Some girls find that before they've quite got over having an orgasm, they can have another one or a series in a row, maybe four or five, with only a few seconds in between. But having a series, or multiple orgasm as it's known, isn't necessarily any better than having one on its own. Most have just the one and that's all they need to feel perfectly satisfied.

All this happens to a girl's body quite naturally when she has an orgasm, whether she's masturbating, practising safer sex which doesn't necessarily involve sexual intercourse, or having intercourse. With all the talk of red flushes and mind-blowing spasms some girls worry that they look very ugly when they come. Nothing could be further from the truth – when does anyone who is feeling excited and happy ever look anything other than lovely? And anyway it doesn't all happen very noticeably to every girl or every time. It doesn't mean she isn't having an orgasm just because her nipples aren't erect, or because her vagina isn't producing much fluid. It's like blushing: some people go red in the face when they're embarrassed, others don't – it doesn't mean that they're any less embarrassed.

Having an orgasm – boys

For a boy the first sign of being sexually aroused is usually an erection. As the sexual excitement increases, his balls swell slightly and draw up close to his body. All his muscles become tense and his breathing gets faster. A warm flush may spread over the front of his body and face. His nipples may become erect and his breasts swell slightly. A few drops of clear fluid (which may have some sperms in it) sometimes come out of the end of his penis.

Inside his body, the sperms are travelling from his testicles to where they are stored for a while at the base of his penis. When the peak of excitement is reached, he feels as if he can't hold back any longer and the sperm comes rushing out along the tube in the middle of his penis and spurts out of the tip in four or five spasms. The spasms spread to all his sex organs, his anus and sometimes the whole of his body. Almost immediately afterwards his penis and the rest of his body relax back to normal.

Can't make it?

There can be many, many reasons why some women find it difficult or seemingly impossible to have an orgasm. The most common reason is that they haven't had enough stimulation. If a girl practises masturbating she'll eventually be able to figure out for herself the amount of stimulation her body needs, and where and how she likes to be touched. It's not always so easy if someone else is doing the stimulating. Intercourse isn't always the best way for the clitoris to be stimulated. And a boy may be so keen to get his penis into her vagina that he doesn't spend enough time arousing her sexually first.

Other reasons for not coming can include being scared of sex, of catching a sexually transmitted disease, or of getting pregnant – especially if you're not using any birth control method. Or it can simply be that you're not in the right mood.

It's easy on the whole for a boy to tell when he's in the mood for sex – he gets an erection. But many girls find it difficult to get aroused if they're thinking about whether someone will come into the room or how uncomfortable and cold it is in the back of a car. Nor is it easy if all she's thinking about is whether or not she'll have an orgasm. You've got to feel relaxed and take the time your body needs to really enjoy sex, and to take pleasure in sex whether you are having an orgasm or not.

Some couples feel they're a complete failure if she doesn't come every single time they have sex. Because of this, some girls like to pretend that they've come when they haven't. With a bit of practice, some heavy breathing, a few writhing movements and some appropriate groans, it's not so difficult to fake. And it may seem like the easy way out if you're being asked insistently if you've come. But there's absolutely no point. For a start, it's nothing more than a lie and a dishonest trick. And if you go on faking you may never learn what it takes for you to have an orgasm. It's usually something that each couple has to work out and, if they can, talk over together. If you've been faking then, when you do want to find out together it's going to be hard to admit that you've been lying for days, weeks, months or maybe years.

Unlike women, men can't have a series of several orgasms in a row. It can take up to several hours before he can have another erection and come again. Usually the younger a boy is the less time it takes. In the space of eight hours some are able to come perhaps six or seven times, others only once or twice. Ignore all claims that a boy has come time after time like some piston engine – he's got to be exaggerating!

Some boys have long-term problems with getting an erection, keeping it up, or in ejaculating. Your doctor may be able to help or tell you where to go for help. Check with your nearest family planning clinic or centre if they have any therapists to help with sex problems like this – you may need to make an appointment and there may be a fee (addresses, page 193). No one can expect a sex therapist to find the automatic cure – but maybe all you need is to talk it over with someone who is understanding. Knowing that you're not the only one with problems is often a great help in itself.

A girl who finds it difficult or impossible to have an orgasm and is upset or worried about it may find that it helps to talk about it with her friends or with other women. Some towns have women's groups which might help with advice or information. Although she or he may not be trained in this field and may even be unsympathetic – especially if you're young – your doctor may be able to help you or send you to a specialist in sex problems. It's worth a try. You can also get help from clinics and centres specializing in sex problems (addresses, page 193). Give them a ring and ask if they have any therapists to advise on sex problems and find out if there is a fee. Sex therapists can't promise an automatic 'cure' – but it often helps to realize that there are people around who don't believe all problems have to last for ever.

Finally: It is important to realize that not everyone has an orgasm every time they masturbate or have sex with a partner. This is perfectly normal and there's no reason why it should be seen as a failure. It can sometimes be very frustrating not to come, but sex isn't just about scoring comes. Having fun, feeling close, getting to know each other and finding out how your and your partner's body works is every bit as important.

CHAPTER SIX

Enjoying Sex

Sex makes a lot of people very happy. There are two parts to how you experience sex – what you do and what you feel in your mind. Feeling good and happy in your mind makes the actual doing a whole lot better. In all relationships it's easy to hurt and be hurt. But perhaps because sex makes people feel so much closer to each other you can probably feel more pain within a sexual relationship than any other sort. Enjoying sex to the full involves a lot of trust and mutual respect, caring, sharing, affection and love between two people.

When we're young, if we have a sex life we usually have to keep it secret. This can make us feel guilty and ashamed of what are, after all, very natural desires and feelings. Many people grow up with a sense of guilt about their sexual feelings. They find it hard to talk openly about sex, they try to hide the fact that they enjoy feeling sexually aroused and, as a result, they may never enjoy sex to the full. What's worse, they sometimes try to prevent others from enjoying sex or knowing anything about it.

At its best, sex can be a way of getting closer to someone you love or care very much about. It's a way of expressing your feelings and of letting your partner know how much you care for them – although it's not the only way. If your partner isn't ready for sex, then you can let them know how much you care by not having sex.

Getting close to someone, or being intimate with them, doesn't only involve sex. It also means being honest and open with them about other things. Then, if there are any problems caused by having sex, you can be more sure that you'll be able to share the problems. For instance, if two people do really care for each other and the girl gets pregnant, or one of you gets a serious disease that can be caught as a result of having sex, or one of you gets into big trouble at home because your parents find out, there'll be someone to turn to for help and support.

It also helps to know something about what you're doing. It's not that there's a right or a wrong way – everybody has their own way of enjoying sex. But there are safe and unsafe ways. The more you know about how to give and get sexual pleasure safely, the more enjoyable and less frightening sex will become.

The best way to relax about sex is to practise safer sex. This means making sure that you don't give or get a disease that you might not even know you have, and making sure that you don't get pregnant. You'll find out more about that on page 62. Of course, the safest way of not getting pregnant or a sexually transmitted disease is not to have sexual inter-course. Safer sex definitely means using a condom plus spermicide if you do have sexual intercourse. Condoms were originally used to stop the spread of serious sexually trans-mitted diseases. But earlier in this century they came to be used mostly as a way of preventing pregnancy. Now we have to use them again to prevent the spread of the virus that causes AIDS. But condoms aren't totally safe. They can break or tear, and then the girl can get pregnant and either partner can get the virus if one of you is infected. Just in case this happens you should also always use a spermicide which contains the chemical Nonoxynol which kills both the virus that can lead to AIDS and sperms on contact. For more about condoms and spermicides see Chapter 8.

This chapter describes some of the ways we can enjoy our own bodies and those of our partner by having sex. If you're not yet ready for a sexual relationship it tells you what to expect and perhaps look forward to if and when you are ready.

Virginity

A virgin is someone – female or male – who has never had sexual intercourse. A lot of very harmful rubbish is talked about virginity. Traditionally it's been thought of as something that a girl should keep at all costs and a boy should lose as soon as possible. Girls were expected to treasure their virginity for when 'Mr Right' came along. But if a boy kept his, he was accused of being immature and 'unmanly'. People like to keep their daughters undersexed and their sons oversexed. Again, fear of pregnancy and lack of information on birth control was part of the reason for this, and attitudes are changing. But many of the myths still exist.

For centuries it's been believed that you can tell if a girl is a virgin by her hymen – the thin membrane that covers the entrance to the vagina. If her hymen was unbroken, then she was a virgin; if it was broken, then she wasn't. And, of course, the only time a girl was expected or permitted to lose her virginity was on her wedding night. This is one reason why girls were told not to masturbate and why mothers advised their daughters against using tampons – Mr Right might turn out not so right if he discovered his blushing bride had a torn hymen!

For a start, many girls are born without a hymen at all. Many hymens have holes in them so it really isn't possible to tell whether it's broken. And many hymens get stretched or broken quite naturally at a young age by riding a bike or horse or by being constipated, without the girl ever knowing.

A girl can find out for herself what state her hymen is in by pushing a finger up her vagina. If it's still in one piece her finger won't go up more than a few centimetres. If her hymen is in one piece the penis makes a hole in it as it enters her vagina when she has intercourse for the first time. Every time she has intercourse after that her hymen gets rubbed down until there's nothing left but a little ring of tissue that often remains round the entrance of her vagina for the rest of her life.

Most hymens are very thin fragile tissues of skin. Breaking this thin skin can sometimes hurt a little. Some girls can feel when it's being broken, and the tiny blood vessels in it may bleed. Most girls dread this happening, but stories about the amount of pain and blood are usually exaggerations. Some girls feel nothing at all and notice no blood. Others may feel a couple of seconds of pain and there'll be a little bleeding – although seldom enough for her to need to use a sanitary towel or tampon.

The most important thing about virginity has nothing to do with whether you have a hymen or not. Everyone is a virgin at some stage of their life and it's important to be honest about it. Having sex for the first time can be difficult enough, both physically and emotionally, without needing the added complication of a lie about whether or not you're a virgin. Being honest can be awkward if you've been pretending that you've done it all before when you haven't, or that you haven't done it when you have. No close relationship, and certainly not a sexual one, is unaffected by starting off with a lie.

Drawing the line

Although attitudes are changing, it's still very widely believed that girls and boys should play entirely different and sometimes totally opposing roles when it comes to sex. Girls often think that they're supposed to pretend not to want or enjoy sex in case they get a 'reputation'. Boys often feel that they're supposed to lead the girl further than she wants to go and live up to some sort of reputation of being randy and sex-mad. Many parents who were brought up to think along these lines tend to be horrified if they discover that their daughter is having sex, but if they discover their son is, they're more likely to think 'good luck to him'.

Having double standards like this can lead to dishonest and very confusing situations. Some girls think they won't be respected if they allow a boy they're really fond of to touch them. Some boys, out of this feeling of respect, find out about sex with a girl they don't really like, but won't touch or share their feelings with a girl they do like. It can be very hard on girls who have to suppress all their sexual feelings and pretend they don't want sex when they do and on girls who, because they do have a sex life, just get labelled as an 'easy lay'. And it can be very hard on boys who aren't sure about what to do or whether they want to have any sex at all if they have to pretend to be super-studs.

One of the most important things that has changed attitudes to sexuality, especially for girls and women, is the enormous increase in knowledge and availability of birth control over the past years – particularly from the 1960s onwards. Being able to have sex without fear of getting pregnant has meant that girls can think of sex as something that they can have for pleasure. And this has changed relations between the sexes too.

Whether you want sex and how far you want to go doesn't depend on whether you are female or male, but on how you feel in yourself as an individual. You may have very good reasons for not wanting a sexual relationship or for wanting to draw the line somewhere. But how other people think you should behave shouldn't be important.

Fear of AIDS may be another reason for not wanting sex or for wanting to draw a line way before intercourse. The safest way to make sure there is no unwanted pregnancy and to prevent AIDS or any other sexually transmitted disease is, of course, to have no sex at all. But this is hardly a helpful suggestion for couples who do want a happy sexual relationship. The solution to this problem is safer sex.

Safer sex

The possibility of getting AIDS is now a danger for everyone whether they're gay or straight, female or male. Sex which involves penetration of the penis into the vagina, anus or mouth is the way in which this disease is spread more than any other way throughout the world.

If you're having sex with a partner who you are absolutely sure doesn't have either the virus that can lead to AIDS or AIDS itself, then you don't have to practise safer sex. But it's not so easy to be absolutely sure. There may be no symptoms at all – your partner may not know if they have the virus. And not everyone is always completely honest with their partners. When people are embarrassed or shy or feel guilty about something they've done, they don't always tell the truth. It is quite possible that your partner really is in love with you, but one night when they weren't with you they may have just happened to have gone to bed with someone else. It happens. They might now feel that it was all a terrible mistake and wish they hadn't. But, rather than tell you and suffer from your anger, or jealousy, they may decide not to tell you. It's not very brave of them (perhaps they think your relationship can't take it), but not everyone is very brave. The trouble is, of course, that they may have got the virus that can lead to AIDS on that night. And if you don't practise safer sex, you might get it too.

Safer sex definitely means using a condom plus spermicide. Condoms don't have to be as bad as some people make out. Millions of couples use them in order not to get pregnant and enjoy a good sex life. But sex doesn't have to mean only penetration.

There's no part of our bodies that can't play a part in enjoying sex. Sexual excitement builds up in each person in different ways through touch, smell, taste and sight. Those areas of our bodies that make us feel sexually aroused when they're touched, stroked or kissed are called erogenous (pronounced with a soft 'g' as in gerbil) zones.

The mouth, lips and tongue of most people are highly erogenous – that's to say kissing can be a turn on. A simple kiss runs no risk of AIDS. Very small traces of the virus have been found in saliva but the experts don't think that kissing is dangerous. French kissing, when you part your lips and let your tongue play with the teeth, tongue and inside of your partner's mouth, may be a bit risky. This is not only because of the saliva that passes between mouths but because it's possible that there might be some blood in the saliva from a sore or a small cut, perhaps caused by some over-strenuous flossing of the teeth. And blood in an infected person does contain high amounts of the virus.

But mouths aren't the only places to kiss. Many girls, and some boys, find it exciting to have their breasts and nipples stroked and kissed. Nipples are very sensitive and become firm and erect when we're sexually aroused. Some people – girls and boys – can have an orgasm just by touching their nipples or by having them touched.

The pleasures of touching, caressing and stroking are often greatly underestimated. You can get to know your own body and that of your partner through gentle caresses, and you can find out what turns you both on. Rubbing or massaging your partner's body with oil – there are lots of lovely smelling oils available these days, but baby oil will do perfectly well – can be very exciting. Taking baths and showers together can be fun too.

The tastes and smell of our bodies can be very exciting, although not everyone realizes this and many people are a bit scared of what they taste and smell like. Undoubtedly, if someone doesn't wash regularly, licking and kissing their body can be bad news – just as bad breath doesn't make a kiss all that wonderful.

There are manufacturers who take advantage of the shyness many of us feel about how we smell. Adverts encourage us to drown our bodies with perfumes and deodorants. Some girls get to feel that they're not properly dressed until they've used their vaginal or underarm deodorant. Vaginal deodorants can in fact cause infections in the vagina and be positively harmful. But in any case, smelling like a plastic geranium isn't much of a turn-on – except maybe to another plastic geranium. And nothing can be more of a turn-off than getting a mouthful of what tastes like disinfectant. All that's needed is regular washing – water comes a lot cheaper than aerosol cans.

The most powerful feelings come from having our genitals gently played with. The heads of the clitoris and penis

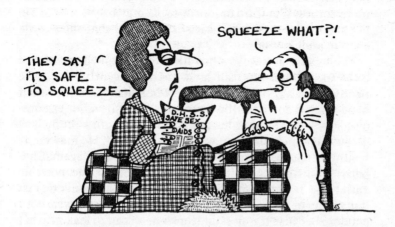

Safer sex means learning lots of new and different ways of enjoying sex.

(especially where the shaft of the penis joins the top) are especially sensitive and stroking just here can easily lead to an orgasm. How we like to be touched varies from person to person. Some girls like their clitoris to be stroked gently, others prefer a bit more pressure. The best way to find out is to ask, or suggest she shows how she likes it.

She may like her partner to give her a come by having the inside of her vagina stimulated with his finger or fingers. This is known as finger fucking. When she's sexually aroused the opening to the vagina usually becomes moist and relaxed and he should find it easy to slide a finger or two gently inside and move them in and out. If her vagina is a bit dry or tense, a little baby oil or some lubricating jelly – you can buy tubes of something called KY Jelly from the chemist – helps. It's best to start off slowly and then begin to speed up a bit. It may be nice for her if he also feels her clitoris or the area around it with his fingers – or she may prefer to do this herself.

After she's come, her clitoris may feel very sensitive and almost too painful to be touched any more. Or she may like her partner to go on stroking her clitoris and will have a few more comes. The third or fourth come may be the best of all, but she may feel perfectly satisfied and feel that she's come enough after just one.

There are many ways a boy likes to be stroked in order to have an orgasm. She can hold his penis gently, but quite firmly, with her fingers or in her whole hand and move her hand up and down, pulling the foreskin (if he's not circumcised) over the head of his penis. Boys who are circumcised get just as much pleasure as those who aren't. He may enjoy feeling her breasts around his penis, or rubbing against her belly, or in her armpit – there's no end to the possible variations. It's not a good idea for him to rub his penis against her vagina or between her closed thighs if he isn't wearing a condom because it is possible for some sperm to leak into her vagina and this could make her pregant or transmit a disease if either partner is infected.

There are various sex toys for couples who want to experiment further. You can buy amazing-looking bobbly condoms and rings that slip over the penis with feathers or little wotsits that are supposed to tickle the clitoris, as well as vibrators and dildoes that some girls and women enjoy being pushed into their vagina. These toys are usually expensive and seldom live up to the wild claims of the manufacturers who are, after all, just in it for the money. But they can be fun or a bit of a lark. Safer sex means that they should only ever be used by one person, never shared, and always kept very clean. Many couples find that honey or yoghurt in some odd place on the body gives just as much fun for a lot less cost.

No two people enjoy sex in exactly the same way, or in the same way each time they have sex. Sometimes she may prefer to make all the movements herself, at other times she may like him to do it all. Likewise, he may want to take all the initiatives, at other times he may prefer her to. The best way to find out how your partner likes sex and what turns her or him on is to talk about it. And talking about sex can be a big turn-on in itself.

Not everyone needs to have an orgasm every time they get aroused or have sex, but learning how to give each other a come by touching, massaging and stroking is a way of having sex which carries absolutely no risk of getting pregnant or of transmitting any disease. (For more about AIDS and safer sex, see page 160.)

Unsafe sex

By experimenting, most couples can find out what they like to do with each other to get and give pleasure safely. It may take a little time to find out and it's easy to feel a bit unsure and awkward at first. Because of AIDS – unless you are absolutely sure that your partner is not infected – you have to be careful of anything that involves blood or semen passing from one body to another. Neither oral nor anal sex is part of safer sex.

Oral sex means using your mouth to enjoy sex by sucking and kissing each other's genitals. Slang words for it include giving head, a blow job and going down. You definitely can't get pregnant by oral sex, but it is risky if you or your partner has AIDS or the virus that can cause AIDS. Another infection called herpes can be transmitted by oral sex.

In oral sex, he kneels down between her legs and feels her clitoris with his tongue. By licking and gently nibbling her clitoris, and maybe poking his tongue into her vagina, he can give her an orgasm. The technical term for this is cunnilingus.

When she goes down on him and gives him an orgasm by licking, kissing or sucking on his penis, it's called fellatio (pronounced fell-art-io). There's nothing poisonous about getting semen in her mouth or swallowing it if she wants to. There's no way in which she can get pregnant from fellatio, but there may be a risk to her of AIDS if he is infected and if she has any sores or cuts in her mouth. The natural acid in the stomach probably kills the virus that can cause AIDS.

When a couple lie on top of each other, or on their sides, and suck each other off, it's called position 69 – presumably because this is what it looks like. It's also called *soixante-neuf*, which is French for 69 (although it's certainly not something that only French couples do).

Some couples enjoy it if he puts his penis inside her anus. This is called anal intercourse or buggery or sodomy. (It is in fact illegal between heterosexual couples, but not between homosexuals.) Unless the anus and penis are well lubricated this can be painful. After the penis has been inside it should be washed as lots of germs live inside the back passage. Anal intercourse is definitely not a part of safer sex because the inside of the anus, being fairly tight and fragile, is likely to tear and bleed a bit. This makes it very easy for infection to pass from any semen directly into the bloodstream, or any blood from an infected person's anus to enter the delicate membranes of the penis.

Intercourse

There are so many expressions for sexual intercourse that it's almost impossible to keep track. The technical words are coitus (pronounced co-ee-tus) and copulation, but they're usually only used by doctors and biology teachers. To make love, to fuck, to lay, to screw, to shag, to have it off or away, to ball, to poke, to shaft, to sleep with, to go to bed with someone and to get your end away are all expressions for the same thing.

The trouble with some of these phrases is that they suggest that intercourse is something that a man does *to* a woman: that the man is the active partner while the woman just lies back and has it all done to her. A man fucks, a woman gets fucked. He screws, she gets screwed. He lays her, she gets laid. Our great-grandmothers were told, 'Lie on your back and think of Queen and country.' It was probably all the sex education they ever got! So women were brought up to think that *because* they were women they had to be passive and let the man do everything. Men were brought up to think that *because* they were men they had to take all the initiatives and not worry too much about whether the woman was getting any enjoyment from sex – because women weren't really expected to enjoy sex.

'Sex is the price women pay for marriage,' went another silly saying, 'and marriage is the price men pay for sex.' Today there are still many people who believe that women and girls have a lower sex drive than men, which partly explains why words like fuck, screw or lay are seldom used to describe what a female does. But sex doesn't mean one thing for women and something totally different and opposite for men. The important thing for each one of us is to find out for ourselves what we like, regardless of our sex. Fucking, screwing and laying are all things that females and males do *with* each other, not what he does to her.

Petting, kissing, hugging, caressing and all the other safe and loving ways of enjoying safer sex are sometimes called foreplay. This suggests that it isn't enjoyable or exciting in itself – which it is. It also suggests that all sex *has* to end in sexual intercourse – which it doesn't. Intercourse is only one way of enjoying sex. Which isn't to say that sexual intercourse is not pleasurable. Without a condom and spermicide it certainly isn't safe: it's one of the easiest way of getting pregnant and of passing on the virus which can cause AIDS.

A lot of people think that condoms are a real turn-off. But they needn't be. In fact, some couples who decide to use them find that putting them on and involving them in their love-making can be exciting. They're certainly cheaper than a lot of other sex toys on the market. All the different colours condoms can be bought in add a bit of fun too.

If a couple does decide to have intercourse it is important that their bodies are ready for it – as well as their minds. Kissing, stroking and touching beforehand relaxes the body and so her vagina will probably produce the natural juices that make it easier for the penis to slip into it. The outer lips will separate as she becomes sexually aroused and the clitoris will poke out of its hood making it easier for it to be stimulated. For him, becoming sexually aroused means that his penis becomes hard and erect in order to push into her vagina.

The reason it doesn't matter whether a penis is long or short, fat or thin, is that when a girl or woman is sexually aroused the innermost part of the vagina stretches to whatever length the penis is. It also has very few nerve endings right up inside so it's difficult for her to feel it very well. The walls of the vagina near the entrance, which do have nerve endings, swell and hug the penis whatever its width.

Many girls fear that their vaginas will get too wide if they have 'too much' sex. In fact, because of the way in which the outermost walls swell, it doesn't matter what size the vagina is. Jokes about cocks so small that they waggle about inside and cunts so slack that cocks get lost aren't very helpful and shouldn't be taken seriously. Most penises and vaginas are more or less the same size.

When the penis goes into the vagina, it's usually best for it to enter gradually with small thrusts rather than one big plunge – the vagina may take a little time before it expands inside. Either partner can help guide the penis in by holding the lips of her vagina apart and finding the entrance with their finger.

To help give the penis the right stimulation and to give the clitoris as much stimulation as possible you need to move rhythmically from your hips so that the penis slides back and forth inside the vagina.

When the penis slides in and out, the lips of the vagina get pulled too. This can have the effect of pulling the hood of skin back and forth over the head of the clitoris, and so may give it all the rubbing and stimulation it needs. Your movements get faster until one of you comes. If she comes first, she can usually go on moving her hips in thrusting movements until he comes and this may add to her pleasure. But if he comes first, his penis goes limp immediately afterwards and he won't be able to give her clitoris any more stimulation except

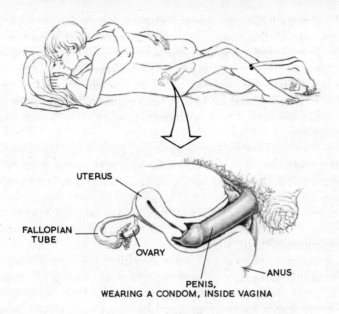

UTERUS

FALLOPIAN
TUBE

OVARY

ANUS

PENIS,
WEARING A CONDOM, INSIDE VAGINA

**This drawing shows a couple making love in the so-called
'missionary' position – but there are lots of other positions.**

with his hand or perhaps by rubbing his genitals against hers.

Many couples are convinced that the only way to enjoy intercourse 'properly' is to come together, having an orgasm at exactly the same time. In fact this rarely happens. And if it does, it isn't necessarily the great thing some people make it out to be. It's fine if you like it. But if you're so involved in your own orgasm, you might not get the rather special pleasure of seeing your partner come. There's no such thing as a 'proper' way to have sex. Whether you come or not, or precisely when you come, is not nearly as important as how you're feeling and how much you enjoy it.

POSITIONS

There are any number of positions a couple can try. The one most often used in this part of the world is called the missionary position. (When European missionaries went to 'heathen' lands, it was they who introduced this position. They were amazed to discover that sex could be enjoyed in other positions, and their would-be converts were amazed to discover that this position could be thought all that enjoyable.) The couple lie looking at each other with him on top of her, she lies on her back with her legs apart, one on each side of his legs.

Some couples never get around to realizing that there's any other way. But it isn't necessarily the best position for her, because it means direct stimulation of her clitoris is impossible. Direct stimulation isn't always necessary, but to help her come in this position it may be a good idea to push a pillow or cushion under her bottom and for her to wrap her legs right round his hips.

If the girl sits on top of the man while he lies on his back, she may find it easier to have an orgasm, as either partner can use their fingers to stimulate her clitoris. Both these positions are nice for couples who like to see each other come. The girl can kneel forward on her hands and knees (often called 'doggy-fashion') or can prop herself up on her elbows and the boy can push his penis into her vagina from behind. Or both can lie on their sides in a 'question marks' or 'spoons' position while he enters her from behind. In any position that the boy enters from behind, the girl will probably need to have her clitoris stimulated with a hand.

If you're disabled, intercourse may be difficult or even impossible. But many disabled people find ways of enjoying sex. An organization called Sexual Problems of the Disabled (SPOD) will give you help if you need it (see page 193).

You can have intercourse standing up (knee-tremblers), sitting down, hanging over the end of the bed, with the girl sitting on a table (table-enders) or chair. Some couples like to try a variety of positions before they come, others prefer to stick to one. Some people like sex in silence, others like to whisper, talk, laugh, cry or shout. Many like sex in a quiet spot in the open air, others like to be in bed. Some like it in the dark, others want the lights on. There are couples who like to be alone and those who enjoy sex with a group of people. But morning or evening, daytime or night time, inside or outside – there's no place, position, time or variation that hasn't been tried or enjoyed (although it's extremely doubtful that anyone *has* ever done it hanging from a chandelier).

Whatever a couple decide to do, whatever variations they hit upon, if both enjoy doing it and find it exciting and satisfying, it's not going to harm anyone. Common sense should tell you if something is dangerous. A good rule of thumb is not to do to anyone else what you wouldn't like them to do to you. Some things may feel new, strange or even peculiar. Don't do them if you don't want to – but you can bet your life it's all been done before. It isn't perverted, abnormal or sick if the aim behind it is to *share* pleasure and if you know you're being careful with someone else's feelings.

THE FIRST TIME – AND AFTER

Some girls find that having intercourse for the first time is so painful or scary that they think they'll never want to try it again. But most find that the second, third, fourth times and so on are a great improvement on the first. Just being scared can make it hurt all the more because you feel so tense when you're scared. You need to relax to enjoy sex. Feeling scared that you'll get pregnant, get a sexually transmitted disease or be found out only makes it all the more difficult.

Feeling very nervous can sometimes make the muscles in the entrance to the vagina close up very tightly, making intercourse impossible. It's only natural for this to happen the first few times. Trying to push on regardless only makes matters worse. If this happens every time and prevents her from ever having intercourse she may need to see a sex therapist to try to sort out the problem.

Some girls find that it hurts every time they have intercourse. This often happens if she has sex just before or during her period when the womb and cervix can be a little tender. Changing to a position in which the vagina gets a chance to stretch out fully – perhaps to the missionary position – will often solve this problem. But the pain could be due to an infection. Even if there is no discharge (the usual sign of an infection) the possibility should be checked out with a doctor (see page 157).

Ignore the myth that people look different after they've had intercourse for the first time. There's no way of telling whether a girl has had intercourse just by looking at her face or by the way she walks. She may feel some soreness in her vagina, but that's all. This is perfectly normal – the vagina won't have had anything as big as a penis in it before. The soreness goes away after a day or two.

If the vagina is dry or doesn't seem to be producing much fluid of its own, intercourse can be fairly painful for both partners. Most often this is due to trying to have intercourse before she has been aroused enough – and if she doesn't get enough stimulation she won't be able to have an orgasm. But the vagina doesn't always produce enough of its own lubrication. A spermicidal jelly or cream is a good way of getting the slipperiness you need. A special sterile lubricating jelly called KY Jelly that can be bought from a chemist will also do the trick. Or a lubricated condom may solve the problem. You'll probably find something around the house like baby oil which will also do. Don't use petroleum jelly if you're using a condom as it tends to rot the rubber. If all else fails, spit will do. Don't worry if your vagina makes a farting noise – this often happens.

Many girls get accused of being frigid or cold if they don't want sex, don't seem to enjoy it, if their vaginas don't produce much fluid or if they never have an orgasm. If on the other hand they do want sex or obviously enjoy it a lot, they get called nymphomaniacs. Calling a girl either of these names is very unfair, for if she does have a minor problem to do with sex, it'll just make her worry and suffer all the more. If she's not enjoying sex to the full, the chances are it's simply because she's feeling nervous. Or it could just mean that she doesn't want sex at that particular time or with that particular person.

Boys who don't seem to want or enjoy sex often think that

they're homosexual or are 'undersexed'. The same can be true for a boy as for a girl – he might just not be wanting sex or he may be wanting it at some other time or with some other person. Sex isn't going to be good or very easy for anyone who doesn't feel like it – and no one feels like it all the time or with everyone.

Many boys find that when they have intercourse for the first time they come very quickly indeed, often even before they've had time to get their penis inside the vagina. This is usually nothing more than a simple case of first-time nerves and it needn't matter too much. Most find that they can get another erection quite quickly. Some will find, however, that this happens every time they have sex – men can get bouts of this problem throughout their lives. Doctors call it premature ejaculation. Some find that the problem is solved by giving themselves a come before they have sex – this makes sure that the sexual excitement builds up more slowly when they're with their partner.

Some boys and men suffer from precisely the opposite problem – they can't get an erection or ejaculation however much they want to. Like coming too soon, it's often due to nerves. Some people believe that using a condom can make the penis go limp. If this always seem to happen, it's worth keeping on trying as condoms are a part of safer sex. And putting them on together involves a lot of stroking and touching and can be very sexy. They can all be part of the fun. His partner may be able to help him keep his erection by holding the base of the penis quite firmly (but not so tightly that it hurts him) between the fingers to prevent the blood from flowing out of the penis – which is what happens when it goes limp. Or she can try squeezing the limp penis into her vagina with her fingers – quite often the penis will grow erect again and they can carry on as if nothing happened. But check that the condom is still on properly. See page 114 for how to put a condom on correctly.

One of the best ways to solve any sex problem is to talk it over with your sex partner. Sympathy, understanding, discovering together possible reasons for the problem and looking for possible solutions could be all that's needed. But if any problem lasts for a time and doesn't seem to be due to first-time nerves or inexperience, don't just sit there – you can do something. The more you worry and bottle up your fears, the worse the problem will become. Go to your doctor if you think she or he will be sympathetic. Some birth control clinics have doctors specially trained to help people with their sex problems (addresses, page 193). Give the clinic a ring first to see if they can help, whether you need an appointment and whether there will be a fee. These clinics and centres will be sympathetic to girls and boys under 16.

Sex aids

Sex shops and surgical stores sell a variety of goods that couples can use when they're having sex. Many of these, often very expensive, are supposed to help people who have difficulties when having sex. There are creams and potions which, the manufacturers claim, will make you and your partner rampant and really wild. It's extremely doubtful that they can have any such effect. Most of the creams which are supposed to keep a penis erect for hours or make a girl come have, when analysed, little more than oil, water and perfume in them. But they don't do any harm and many people are so convinced that they work that they *do* have some effect. There are condoms with rubber knobs sticking out all over them which are supposed to give a girl feelings of ecstasy. This is doubtful, but, as one doctor has said, if you enjoy looking at a randy sea anemone, it can be money well spent. One warning here – don't use these condoms as a method of preventing pregnancy or of catching a disease without checking – condoms are only reliable if they carry the British Safety Standards kitemark on them.

APHRODISIACS

Aphrodisiacs are substances which supposedly make you feel

more sexy. For someone who thinks they have a low sex drive or who has difficulty in getting in the right mood for sex they sound like an answer to a prayer. But in fact there's no such thing as an aphrodisiac. In the past, tomatoes, potatoes, peppers, oysters, musk, powdered rhino horn, seaweed and countless other things have all been thought to have magical powers to make people feel sexy. It is of course true that if we don't eat a good balanced diet we feel less like sex than if we eat fresh healthy foods. But there's no food or drug which can actually make us sexually aroused. A warning about a substance called Spanish Fly. This is a powder made from crushing the bodies of certain beetles which many people believe to be an aphrodisiac. Swallowing Spanish Fly is highly dangerous. It is a poison which can cause – and has caused – death.

Although many sex aids and toys can be fun, they're sold in their tons to people who actually think that they'll cure their sex problems. In fact what they mostly do is to make their manufacturers very rich.

DRUGS

People take drugs for a variety of reasons – for fun, to relieve boredom, because they're depressed, for curiosity or because they think that drugs can increase the pleasure of sex. The myths that surround drug-taking are, like all myths, not very reliable.

Drugs don't and can't affect our sex organs. Some, it is true, can lower our inhibitions, relax our muscles and increase our awareness of our bodies to a certain extent. But no two people react in the same way to any one drug. Some drugs can make some people feel good but they can make others feel tensed up, sick and turn them completely off sex.

Unlike sex, drugs are not something that our bodies need naturally. Some drugs are positively dangerous, others are less so. The pleasure we can get from sex depends on how you feel about your sex partner and not on what drugs you take.

Injecting drugs into your bloodstream (called IV drug use, short for IntraVenous, which means into the veins) does nothing whatsoever for your sex life, and it is one of the main ways in which the virus that causes AIDS can be transmitted. For more information about this, see page 160.

ALCOHOL

Alcohol is a drug which can and does cause just as much physical and mental harm as many drugs which are illegal or available only on prescription.

It is generally believed that alcohol increases the sex drive – 'Three martinis and she's anyone's' being the generally accepted rule of thumb. Drinking a little can lower our inhibitions to make us feel less shy, but basically alcohol is a depressant. The main problem with alcohol is that it only requires a small amount to stop people from thinking too clearly. This makes it easy to go on drinking and become really drunk and ill. Too much alcohol will make you feel sleepy, put you off sex and make it difficult to have an orgasm. It has the unhappy effect of making us feel randy but decreasing the quality (or likelihood) of performance. Many boys find that once they're drunk they can't get an erection – 'brewer's, or drinker's, droop' as it's often called.

Despite the havoc and unhappiness that alcohol can cause, it's a socially acceptable drug. But like drugs, whether legal or illegal, it's the manufacturers and sellers who profit in the end.

Under 16?

A man or boy commits a crime if he has sexual intercourse with a girl who is under the age of consent. In England, Scotland and Wales, this age is 16. In Northern Ireland and the Republic of Ireland it is 17. It doesn't matter whether or not the girl agreed and wanted to have intercourse. The girl doesn't commit a crime. The term 'age of consent' refers to the age when a girl is considered by the law to be old enough to agree to have sexual intercourse.

In practice the law works as follows:

—*If he is under 14* he can't be prosecuted.

—*If she is under 13* and he is over 14, it's a serious crime. He won't be able to defend himself by claiming he thought she was older.

—*If he is under 24* and she is between 13 and 15, he may be able to claim in court that he thought she was older.

—*If he is over 24*, the risk of prosecution and conviction increases.

Sentences vary greatly. If the boy is under 17 he won't be sent to prison but he may be placed in the care of the local authority. If he is over 17 he can get up to two years in prison. If the girl is under 13 the sentence could mean life (twenty-five years).

A woman or girl can't be accused of unlawful sexual intercourse. But if the boy is under 16 she can be found guilty of indecent assault which carries a penalty of up to two years' imprisonment.

For a boy to be taken to court for unlawful sexual intercourse, a complaint has to be made to the police. This can be made by anyone – it's usually made by the girl's parents. The police then decide whether or not to go ahead with the prosecution. Because this law is thought by many people to be very unfair (why should boys or men be prosecuted but not girls? Does it make sense for it to be illegal to have sex on the day before her sixteenth birthday but not at one minute past midnight on her birthday?), quite often the police decide not to prosecute.

A boy who finds himself taken to court for unlawful sexual intercourse will need a solicitor (see page 187). A girl under 16 who is – or thinks she is – pregnant, or has a sexually transmitted disease, may find herself under some pressure to reveal the name of the boy involved. It's very unlikely for a doctor or social worker to make a complaint to the police, but this has happened. If she wants to protect the boy from the law she'll have to refuse to give his name. But if she does this she might be accused of having sex with so many boys that she doesn't know who the father is; if she is thought to be 'promiscuous', if her parents, teacher, police or social worker think that she is in 'moral danger', she could find herself in court and put into the care of the local authority, even though she has not broken the law.

CHAPTER SEVEN

The Misuse and Abuse of Sex

Sex is a lot more than just a set of cold facts about what parts of the body go where. A simple 'how to do it' approach ignores that sex and our sexual feelings are about the whole of our bodies and our minds: our feelings about ourselves and about how we relate to others, our values and how we value ourselves. When it's good, sex is a part of loving someone. It means listening to the other person and considering their needs as well as your own.

Sex is often misused in our society. Different people have different ideas about what is meant by the misuse of sex. Some families believe that all sex outside marriage is a misuse. Others believe that if there is mutual caring and sharing, then sex is acceptable. Neither way of thinking is right or wrong. Each one of us has to work out what is right or wrong for ourself.

But there are some ways in which sex is used which are definitely wrong. Any unequal relationship where one partner doesn't say yes to sex of their own free will can never be right. Rape, sexual harassment and other forms of sexual abuse involve a more powerful person imposing their need for some sort of sexual satisfaction over and above the needs of the other.

The sexual abuse of children and young people has gone on since time began. Possibly because it was so frightening it wasn't often talked about. The victims of abuse were usually ignored and not believed. But it's beginning to come out into the open because those who were abused when they were children – mostly girls – refused to be shut up about it any longer.

Incest and abuse of care

By law we are not allowed to marry or have sexual relations with our mother, father, step-parent, grandmother or grandfather, sister or brother, uncle or aunt. Sexual intercourse (in either the vagina or the anus) with anyone from this list is called incest. Other forms of sexual abuse include the touching of genitals and oral sex with anyone from this list. The law also protects young people from sexual relationships with adults whose job it is to look after them, such as a guardian, foster-parent, teacher, member of staff of a children's home, a parent's live-in lover, etc. This is called abuse of care.

Incest and abuse of care happen in every kind of family – rich and poor, upper-, middle- and working-class, white and black, and people from all religions. The most common form of incest takes place between a father or stepfather and daughter or stepdaughter. It can happen at any age. It may be just one incident or it may go on for years.

It is extremely difficult for any child or young person to prevent it from happening. Sometimes they're far too young even to realize that it's a form of abuse. We're all brought up to think that our elders are our betters and to do what we're told. An abuser relies on this to sexually abuse a child. And apart from this, any adult or older relative is a lot bigger and stronger than a child. The abuser may use actual physical force to make the child have sex, or they may use a more subtle form of threat or persuasion, such as 'I'll go to prison if you tell and it'll be your fault for splitting up the family', or 'You'll break your mother's heart if you say anything.' Or they may bribe a child by offering a present or telling them that they won't be loved if they don't do it.

Incest and abuse of care can be totally horrifying. A child feels stuck and doesn't know how to get out of the situation.

Sometimes it can also be pleasurable. Some victims of incest and sexual abuse feel guilty about it because they either got some enjoyment out of it, or because they took an active part in it.

However it happened or whatever took place it is *always* the older person who is responsible for committing the crime. To a certain extent our bodies react to being touched a bit automatically and outside our total control. Any pleasurable feelings we get from having our genitals touched is quite normal, even if we know that the person doing the touching shouldn't be doing it. And quite often, if this happens when we're very young, we don't know that it shouldn't be happening. If we love the person – father, grandparent or whoever – it's obviously especially difficult to tell whether what happens should be taking place.

TELLING

Most people who have suffered from incest find it incredibly difficult to tell anyone – even when they're much older. They are frightened that the abuser will try to get some awful revenge, that they will be blamed for splitting up the family or that they simply won't be believed. Or someone who has been abused may feel incredibly guilty and think that it's their fault.

It is important to tell someone. And to go on trying to tell until you find someone who will believe you. If this has happened to you – even if it was a long time ago when you were very young – you should find someone to tell. People who have been sexually abused when they were children all say that the experience affects the way they think about themselves, about sex, and their relationships in adult life. The fears and problems suffered by an incest victim almost never just fade away.

It is getting easier for those who have been abused to speak out and to be believed. There are several help organizations that you can contact if you have been abused in this way. They are listed on page 198. They will be sympathetic and treat all you have to say in confidence. You can also phone the social services department (look in the phone book under the name of your local authority) and ask to speak to the duty social worker.

Remember: it was NOT your fault. Incest, abuse of care and any type of sexual abuse done to a young person is a crime committed by the older person who took advantage of the age and possibly muddled feelings of the child. (In law, a child or young person is anyone under the age of 16.)

Rape

When a man forces a girl or woman to have sexual intercourse and forces his penis into her vagina or anus, it is called rape. Boys can be raped if a boy or man forces him to have anal intercourse. The vast majority of rapes take place between male rapists and female victims.

Most people probably think that a rapist is a weird and nasty stranger who attacks their victims on deserted moors or in parks or jumps out from alleyways late at night. This is why most young children – especially girls – are told not to be out late at night or be on their own in deserted places, and never to talk to strangers. In fact, most rapists are men who are known to the girls and women they rape. This is called acquaintance rape. If you think about it, this means that most rapists are men who seem to be perfectly friendly, normal men whom you would never dream would be rapists. Most teenagers are raped by someone they know and trust, often about the same age. A boyfriend, perhaps, or a friend of a friend, someone they met at a party, or whom they half know, such as an assistant in a shop they go to, or a neighbour. The rapist seldom attacks his victim suddenly out of the blue from behind a bush but usually uses the fact that his victim knows or half knows him, and the rape happens gradually, often in a place where the teenager assumes she will be safe. Because so-called 'nice boys' are usually involved, acquaintance rape is often taken less seriously than rape by a stranger. But rape is a serious crime whoever does it.

There is often a suspicion in people's minds that it is impossible for a woman or girl to be raped: that if she really didn't want it, she would be able to resist in some way. Many films and books (usually made or written by men) suggest that women actually enjoy the experience of being treated roughly and having a strong man forcing himself upon her. The confusion here is between the fantasy of rape and the reality. There is literally nothing that the human mind can't fantasize about. And there's no harm in imagining or fantasizing about being treated roughly and dragged off by some strong handsome man who wants sex with you. But the reality is very different from any fantasy. Fantasy doesn't harm anyone. The reality of rape most certainly does.

And then there's a double standard which suggests that a girl or woman 'asked' for it by her manner or the clothes she was wearing. Men and boys, of course, can wear what they like, walk where they like and behave how they like without people assuming that they want to be sexually abused or raped. A girl or woman who does flirt with a man, who walks home alone, or who wears sexy clothes isn't asking to be raped: she's only wanting a good time, wanting to feel attractive or wanting to get home. She may be a bit silly to do any of these things – but she does not deserve to be raped merely for being silly.

Rape is a truly awful crime and no girl or woman ever wants to be raped. She *never* asks for it. Anyone who has been raped or has read about it would realize this immediately. Firstly, it's very frightening to have a boy or man, usually stronger than yourself, force sex upon you by threatening perhaps to kill or disfigure you if you refuse. You can't just cross your legs and tell the rapist to go away. Also, rape often involves being peed on, shat on, spat on, and/or hit, as well as the sexual assault. And quite apart from all these things, it doesn't take much imagination to realize how awful it is simply to be treated not as a person who is valued and loved or cared for, but simply as a thing with a vagina.

IF YOU ARE RAPED – SOME GUIDELINES

Try to stay as calm as you can. If you think you might be badly hurt, try not to struggle. Say, if you can, that you don't want sex – or words like that. Sometimes it's such a frightening experience that girls and women find that they can't say anything at all. But if you can, it's a good idea to try to talk yourself out of the situation. You can try asking how he would feel if this happened to his mother, sister or girlfriend. Crying, screaming or peeing can put the rapist off. Or you can pretend you are pregnant, have your period or even that you have a disease that he might catch.

There aren't any sure ways of stopping the rapist. Most women who have been raped say that it's best to trust your own instincts during an attack. The most important thing is to stay alive. And if you think that your screaming might make him even more violent – then don't scream.

DO YOU REPORT A RAPE?

Contact a friend, parent or someone you trust. For girls and women, there are several Rape Crisis Centres which will help and give you moral support. Or try to find someone to go with you to the police station if you decide to report it. If you are a heterosexual boy who has been raped, you will have to call on your friends or family for help and support. If you are gay, you can ask for help from one of the gay switchboard organizations in your area (see page 198).

In principle it's a good idea to report the rape to the police. This might discourage some rapists who get away with it and do it again. But you have to be brave to report it. Very often, the ordeal that you go through once you have reported it is so unpleasant that it's understandable why many women prefer to keep quiet about it. In court, the man's lawyer may try to make out a case that the woman is immoral or promiscuous, that she led him on, that because she didn't struggle she's lying about being raped – and many other nasty accusations. You can be asked many searching questions about your

previous sex life, but your name is no longer allowed to be
published in the newspapers.

REPORTING IT TO THE POLICE

—Tell the police as soon as possible; delay may go against
 your case.
—If you can, tell someone what has happened – you may need
 a witness to your distress.
—Don't wash, tidy yourself up or change your clothing; you
 may destroy valuable evidence. Don't have a bath, because
 if there is any semen this will be used in evidence.
—Don't take any alcohol or drugs.
—Contact a friend, your parents or a Rape Crisis Centre
 (address and number, page 198) so that someone can go
 with you and give you moral support during the police and
 medical procedures.
—Take a change of clothing with you; the police may keep
 some of your original clothing for tests and evidence.
—Be prepared for a medical examination. You can ask for
 your own doctor or a woman doctor to be present.
—You can ask for your name to be withheld.

GETTING OVER THE RAPE

Many people who have been raped say that it is a very difficult
experience to get over quickly. The problem isn't helped by
those sort of people who insist on blaming the victim. This
attitude makes some people who have been raped feel like
victims for the rest of their lives. But many people do come
through it and learn that they are survivors rather than
victims. In order to get back your confidence about yourself,
it really is a very good idea to take the time to talk about your
feelings after you have been raped.

If you are a girl or woman, a Rape Crisis Centre will help. If
there isn't one in your area, give the London one a call to see if
they can put you in touch with one near you. A boy who has
been raped could try telling his doctor (as can any girl or

woman). Some doctors may be unhelpful and merely suggest that you pull your socks up, forget about the experience, and get on with life. But the more helpful and intelligent doctors will realize that it is never this easy. Our minds can play strange tricks on us. Just when we think we've forgotten all about it, the fears and problems can come belting out and stop us from getting on with life. And when something this traumatic has happened, how can we pretend that nothing has happened? Some doctors can put you in touch with a counsellor or therapist you can talk it over with. It isn't just nutty people who go to therapists – their skill is in knowing that people's minds and feelings are very complicated and that no two people react in the same way. They're there to help you, and you'll need some help from a skilled person.

In order to feel more secure and get back your confidence, it's worth taking some practical steps. Make sure you have good locks on your windows and doors. Ask a friend to travel with you rather than run the risk of feeling scared when you're on your own. And you might like to think about joining a self-defence class.

Dirty phone calls

Dirty or obscene phone calls can be very frightening. They're almost always made by a male to a girl or woman. Obviously an obscene phone call doesn't hurt anyone physically – but it can and does cause a lot of mental upset to the person who gets the call. You always think that the caller might know your address and might come round and actually do the things they're talking about on the phone.

In fact, most boys and men who make dirty phone calls are probably fairly lonely people who may be masturbating while they're talking. This may well be because they're too afraid to have a real relationship with a girl or woman. But although they may not be dangerous, it's never nice to feel yourself being treated as just anybody who is merely being used to help a complete stranger jerk off against your ear.

There are some practical ways of dealing with obscene phone calls:

—If a phone caller whose voice you don't recognize tries to get you to give him your name, just put the phone down. If it is a real friend, he'll phone back.

—Don't give either your name or phone number when you answer a call. If he asks you what your number is, just ask 'What number were you calling?' If he doesn't know, put the phone down.

—If you have an answering machine, ask a male friend to do the message for you.

—If you've had a dirty phone call, try to get a male friend to answer the phone for you whenever possible until you feel safe.

—Cut off a dirty phone caller by saying something like 'I'm sorry, this is a bad line, I can't hear you' before putting the phone down. He probably won't bother to phone again if he thinks he can't be heard.

—Buy a really piercing whistle – the kind used for mountain rescue – from a sports shop and blast his ears with it before putting down the phone.

—Tell the police. They can't do much, but they may keep an eye on your house. If the calls go on and on, they may be able to trace the call.

—You can ask British Telecom to intercept your calls. You can give them a list of people who you allow to phone you – they won't put anyone else through.

—If this last idea isn't very practical, you can arrange with British Telecom to change your number. You can also go ex-directory so that your name and number aren't in the phone book.

—Talk it over with someone – either a friend, parent or guardian, or a therapist or counsellor. Obscene phone calls are always disturbing. You may need some help in learning not to think of yourself as a passive victim who gets these unwanted and unasked-for calls.

If you are ever tempted to make a dirty phone call for a joke – don't. To the person getting the call it can be a lot more than just a silly joke. It's an invasion of their privacy and it can be both frightening and upsetting. If you find yourself doing it because you feel you have to and you get a sexual kick out of doing it, you need help. Counsellors and therapists are there to help you as well as your victims. Contact one of the organizations on page 187.

Flashers

Flashers – called exhibitionists – get sexually aroused (or try to) by exposing their genitals to strangers. They're mostly men, although there are also women exhibitionists, who are unable to get sexually aroused in any other way.

For any girl, being exposed to can be very upsetting and it's only natural to feel scared and angry – it's never nice to have an unwanted sexual experience or to be reminded that in our society many people think of women as sex objects. Also young girls aren't always sure what an exhibitionist's intentions are, and can be frightened by this. In fact very few exhibitionists ever want to harm or even touch the person they're exposing themselves to. Most are impotent and unable to get an erection when it comes to close contact with anyone.

Most doctors and sex therapists see exhibitionism as a symptom of a person's inability to relate to other people, but indecent exposure is a crime, and any exhibitionist who is reported to the police and then convicted can get up to three months in prison for a first offence and twelve months for any further convictions.

You may not think it worth reporting a flasher to the police. But some people are very frightened by this type of experience and by telling the police you may be able to prevent another person suffering more badly than you.

If this does happen to you, tell a parent, guardian or friend.

Sharing it with someone you know and trust helps make you feel less upset by it.

Peeping Toms

A peeping Tom is also known as a voyeur, which is the French word for someone who watches. In a sexual sense it means someone who gets sexually aroused by looking at people undressing or having sex. The law usually concerns itself with male voyeurs – but there are some women who do it too. Voyeurs often satisfy their sexual urges by peeping through keyholes, looking through windows or by hanging around public toilets and changing rooms in shops and swimming pools. Voyeurs can be charged with 'insulting behaviour', or 'causing a breach of the peace', which both carry punishments of up to six months' imprisonment.

It can be frightening to be watched, especially if there's someone crawling outside your window or up a tree outside your bedroom. And it's never pleasant to be treated as a sex object. Apart from trying to make sure that you can't be seen (draw the curtains or blind at night) you can also report the incident to the police. Even if it doesn't bother you too much, he may do it to someone else who gets really disturbed by it.

If you are worried about being a voyeur yourself, go to see a sex therapist at a clinic (see page 187 for addresses).

Sexual harassment

There is a wide range of behaviour that counts as sexual harassment. Some people, usually men, get sexual satisfaction from rubbing their penis up against someone else, usually a girl or women, in a public place like a crowded bus, on the underground, at a concert or a football match, etc. They're called *frotteurs*, which is a French word for someone who rubs. Then there are those who get off by touching or brushing up against other people's bottoms or breasts. A milder – but still unpleasant – form of sexual harassment is the sort of whistling or leering, or cheap and nasty sexual remarks, by men when girls and women walk by.

None of these types of behaviour, usually by boys and men, are about treating females as individuals who are respected or cared for. In other words, it reduces a female to no more than sex objects for men to treat however they please – as if they were just dolls or playthings. It has very little to do with sexual attraction: some boys and men will behave in this gross manner to any and every passing female. As one girl put it, it makes her feel like no more than a 'walking vagina'.

If you are sexually harassed at school – either by another pupil or by a teacher – you should report it at once. You may want to talk it over first with a parent or guardian, with your friends, or with a sympathetic teacher. Don't be put off by someone who thinks it's not worth bothering about. It's your body and you have every right to have your body respected. If it bothers you, then it is worth bothering about. And if a mild form of sexual harassment doesn't worry you, it may upset someone else very much indeed. The sort of person who treats you like this is probably doing it to others as well.

If you are sexually harassed in your office or place of work, you can report it to someone who is in a position to stop it. Or you can take legal action. The Citizens Advice Bureau, the National Council for Civil Liberties or a local law centre will tell you what your rights are. If you get sacked as a result of complaining (it may be your boss who is harassing you – it's often done by men who rely on your more junior and therefore weaker position) you can again either consult a lawyer or take it to the Equal Opportunities Commission (see page 188).

Pornography

Pornography is erotic material – books, pictures, films – that makes people feel sexually aroused. 'Soft-core' porn usually means pictures of naked women and men (usually women), very much like the sort of photos you can see every day in newspapers like the *Sun*. 'Girlie' magazines such as *Playboy* and *Penthouse* go a little further in what they describe and show, but they're usually thought to come into the soft-core category. 'Hard-core' porn goes much further and has detailed pictures and descriptions of every sexual activity you can think of, leaving nothing to the imagination.

The law tends to turn a blind eye to soft-core but it does try to ban hard-core pornography from being sent through the post, from being brought into the country and from being sold in shops. Other laws make it a risky business to show pornographic films or 'blue movies' in public cinemas or private clubs.

Pornography and censorship are very controversial issues. There are those who would like to see all porn banned because so much of it does tend to emphasize the crude physical aspects of sexual relationships. Those who argue against censorship believe that the banning of porn can do more harm than the porn itself – that censorship laws make many people feel that it's wrong and depraved to feel sexually aroused, and that sexual satisfaction has therefore to be got 'under cover'.

In fact there's no reliable evidence which proves that looking at and enjoying porn results in sex crimes or crimes of violence. Indeed, there are doctors and sex therapists who give erotic material to patients with sex problems to help them learn how to get sexually aroused.

One of the main problems about porn is that most of it is produced for men by men who just want to make large profits. Because of the kind of society we live in, this means that much of it makes the women look like dumb performing animals or concentrates on pictures which relate sex with violence – which obviously many people find disgusting. A lot of porn confirms the widespread belief that it is enjoyable to treat women as nothing more than sex objects.

Another problem is that it's very difficult, especially if we live in a city, to avoid looking at porn, even if we try. We should all have the right to decide how and when we want to look at erotic material or think about sex, but our daily popular papers, advertising hoardings and posters outside strip clubs, some pubs and cinemas give us very little choice.

Laws which attempt to ban totally all pornography have little effect other than to push up the price of erotic books and films and to make many people feel guilty about their desire to be sexually aroused. Making porn illegal certainly does nothing to change the nature of erotic material. A society in which women were treated more as equals and which was less disapproving of people wanting to be sexually excited would perhaps produce erotic material which didn't rely on material so degrading to women.

The world of porn is a nasty one. Some girls and women who model for pornographic books and magazines undoubtedly get good money. And most find that their bodies are just being used: used to make the publishers rich and the readers horny. The models certainly aren't valued for themselves as people. Most models find that their bodies aren't 'good enough' anyway – most of the photos get retouched and altered simply in order to satisfy the readership. And any girl or women whose picture is available to any and every man who happens to buy a magazine is certainly thought to be available herself to any and every man. Don't be tempted by anyone offering you a 'modelling' job. And don't agree to let anyone photograph you in the nude. It's not worth it.

Prostitution

The large majority of prostitutes are women who agree to have sex with a man for a sum of money. There are also a very small number of men prostitutes who have women clients, and there are gay and bisexual prostitutes. Few women who become prostitutes ever had much choice about their work – the majority needed money and had no other way of earning it. Many of them are exploited by men called ponces or pimps who set them up in business, make it difficult for them to stop working, and who take most of their money off them.

In the UK, prostitution itself isn't exactly illegal, but there are so many offences that can be committed only by a prostitute or by those involved in the organization of prostitution that it might as well be.

Paying for sex won't give either the client or the prostitute any idea of how good a loving, caring and mutually sharing sexual relationship can be. Prostitutes are generally made to feel like sex objects by their clients (think of the way people use the word 'whore'), like criminals by the law and like outcasts by the rest of society. Clients are made to feel as if a natural need for sex is a crime.

In some countries prostitution has been made legal and there are state brothels (a brothel is any building in which prostitutes work). This means that sexually transmitted diseases can be kept in check more easily, that prostitutes can earn a living wage, and that they're not terrorized by their pimps. But although legalized prostitution might be a way of ending some of the more obvious ways in which prostitutes are exploited, it doesn't solve the basic problem – that any sexual relationship which involves the buying and selling of sex has to be an unequal relationship. In a system of nationalized prostitution the role of the pimp has simply been transferred from a private individual to the local council or government.

There are people, women and men, who for a variety of reasons either can't or don't want any emotional involvement in their sexual relationships. Nor do they necessarily want their sex lives to consist entirely of masturbation. Prostitution may help them, but it doesn't solve the important problem of taking advantage of or exploiting someone sexually. But at least if prostitutes didn't have to work on the fringes of the criminal world, as they do in the UK, perhaps fewer prostitutes would be make to feel like criminals and fewer of their clients would be made to feel guilty about their need for sex.

Sex and money are quite closely linked in our society. A lot of adverts suggest that if only you were rich enough you could get the prettiest or sexiest boyfriend or girlfriend in the world.

And a lot of boys and men still think that if they buy a girl or woman a meal, then she owes them sex. Some teenagers get dragged into prostitution because they're desperately in need of money. But it is possible to get out of this mess. Various agencies listed on page 198 can help young people who get into this situation. It's important to get out: the risks are of sexually transmitted diseases, brutal sexual assault, possible future problems in relationships, unwanted pregnancy, and even murder.

Prevention: Some dos and don'ts

Simply saying 'No' when someone is trying to abuse you and to misuse sex, isn't always easy. But there are some dos and don'ts that can help you from getting into a situation where it might happen.

First of all the dos:

—Do make sure that your house or flat, if you live on your own, has good strong locks on doors and windows.
—Do draw curtains and blinds when it's dark.
—Do check out the company if you go for a job interview – especially if it's one advertised on a card in a local newsagent's.
—Do be realistic about the sort of clothes you wear. Obviously no one should be judged by the sort of clothes they wear – but you're not going to change society on your own. It may sound trite, but it really is better to be safe than sorry.
—Do treat other people as you would like to be treated yourself.
—Do make sure you always have enough money for the fare home and the right change to make a phone call should you need to.

And the don'ts:

—Don't be on the lookout merely for strangers. Most rape, all incest and abuse of care, and many forms of sexual harassment are done by people (mostly males) to those (mostly females) who know them. As one writer has pointed out, teaching children only to be wary of strangers is like teaching kids how to cross the road but to look out only for red cars.

—Don't hitchhike – and certainly never on your own.

—Don't give your name or number when answering the phone. And don't ever say that you're alone in the house to someone who might take advantage of this knowledge.

—If someone comes to your door and you have to go back inside in order to get some money or something, shut the door first. You may think this seems rude – but it's not worth taking any risks just in the name of politeness.

—Don't babysit for strangers. And always give the phone number and address of where you're babysitting to someone who can check up if you're all right should you be late.

—Don't babysit with a boyfriend unless you are really sure of him.

—Don't walk around the streets late at night on your own. If you have no other option (you might, for instance, decide to walk home on your own rather than accept a lift from someone you don't trust or you're not sure of), try to act like you're feeling really confident and keep to well-lit streets. Of course everyone, female as well as male, should have the right to walk where and when they want to. But, again, you're not going to change society on your own.

—Don't put any pressure on your boyfriend or girlfriend to have sex unless you feel really sure that they want to.

Finally, some adults are learning that teaching young people to say 'No' isn't enough. We all have to think about changing those attitudes which mean girls are brought up to be weaker and more passive than boys, and boys are encouraged to think that being tough and aggressive is the right way to become men. It's this sort of thinking that leads to the misuse and abuse of sex.

There's a really good book called *Too Close Encounters and What to Do About Them*, by Rosemary Stones (published by Magnet) which tells you all you need to know about the misuses and abuses of sex in much more detail. Every teenager should read it. So should adults – they'd learn that it's *never* the fault of the young person abused.

CHAPTER EIGHT

Birth Control

When a boy ejaculates there are millions of tiny sperms in his semen. It only takes one of these sperms to make a girl pregnant. What happens is this: the sperms swim up the vagina, into the womb and up the fallopian tubes. If any one sperm meets a ripe egg on its way down from an ovary towards the womb it may pierce the wall of the egg and enter it. The egg is then fertilized by the sperm – the process is known as conception. Once this has happened the girl is said to have conceived and she is pregnant. The fertilized egg travels down the fallopian tube and, once in the womb, it settles on the thickened walls of the womb.

Every single time a girl and boy have intercourse a baby may be conceived. The only way of making sure that a girl doesn't get pregnant is, quite simply, not to have intercourse. But if you want to have intercourse and not have a baby, you must use a really reliable method of birth control or contraception. In technical terms, contraception means 'against conception'. In human terms it means that a girl does not get pregnant.

Facts and figures can seem rather unreal, but think of the possible human misery behind these:

—Every year, thousands of girls under the age of twenty are pregnant on their wedding day.

   Did she or her boyfriend really want to get married? Did she – or her partner – want to start marriage with a baby? How did they tell their parents? Do they both earn enough money to really look after the baby?
—Every year thousands of unmarried teenage girls become single parents.

Did her boyfriend just up and leave when he found out he was going to be a father? Is she able to look after her baby and keep a job if she has one? Does she have anywhere for them to live?
—Every year thousands of teenage girls have abortions to end their pregnancy.

How much did this cost? Was she forced into it? Did she have to go through this on her own? Is she feeling sad that she's lost her baby?
—Every year thousands and thousands of girls are scared almost out of their minds because they think they might be pregnant when they don't want to be

It all adds up to an awful lot of misery for a lot of people (mostly girls and women). And it could nearly all be prevented. The answer is: contraception.

Until the late 1960s, it wasn't easy to get advice about contraceptives unless you were married. But today it's a relatively simple matter to find out how you can have sex with virtually no risk of getting pregnant if that's what you want. The methods are free or quite cheap, and easy to use. Though it's more difficult to get contraceptive advice in some parts of the country than others, more and more doctors now realize how important it is that every baby should be a wanted baby, and that the way to prevent unwanted babies from being born is to give people advice about birth control methods. The birth control clinics listed on pages 193–4 are helpful and friendly – they won't worry about your age or whether you're married or unmarried. The clinics and most doctors are there to help – don't take risks.

Every method of birth control involves some thinking and planning in advance. Some people think that preparing for intercourse is cold-blooded and unromantic. If you think that taking the risk of getting pregnant is 'romantic' you should think again, carefully. How much 'romance' is there going to be around if you get pregnant?

Sex can, and often does, 'just happen', but it's not worth chancing it. Unless you think in advance and take precautions, once a sperm gets into the vagina there's nothing you can do but cross your fingers and hope. And hoping never stopped anyone from getting pregnant. It is true that no contraceptive is absolutely foolproof or one hundred per cent safe – but the least safe method is using no contraceptive at all.

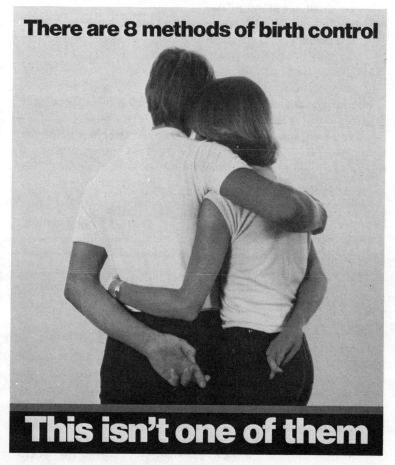

There are 8 methods of birth control

This isn't one of them

Ignore the myths about birth control and never take risks.

The myths

The myths about preventing a pregnancy probably do more harm than any of the other myths about sex. Do NOT believe anyone who claims (or worse, tries to persuade you) that any of the following 'methods' will prevent you from getting pregnant:

—if you have sex standing up
—if she jumps up and down, coughs or sneezes after sex
—if she doesn't have an orgasm
—if he has a hot bath immediately before sex
—if she has a hot bath immediately after sex
—if she pees immediately after sex
—if she washes out her vagina with lemon juice, vinegar, Coca-cola (or anything else) immediately after sex
—if you have sex during, just before or just after her period.

These methods DON'T work, CAN'T work and NEVER worked.

A girl isn't necessarily going to get pregnant every time she has sex without using a contraceptive. This is probably why so many people think that there are definite times of the month when it is 'safe' to have sex without needing to use a contraceptive. But this isn't true – the risk is there every time. Girls have got pregnant by having sex during, before and after their period. And for many girls, getting pregnant happens very easily indeed.

Whose responsibility?

The two most reliable methods of birth control are the pill and the IUD or coil. Unfortunately they're also the ones for which girls and women have to take all the responsibility on their own – although both partners can go along to the birth control clinic to discuss it all together. And neither method is of any use when it comes to safer sex and making sure that neither of you gets a sexually transmitted disease. One of the next most reliable methods is the condom when used with a spermicide, and this is the only method for couples practising safer sex to prevent the possibility of getting the virus that can cause AIDS. Using a condom on its own is not one hundred per cent certain to prevent either pregnancy or disease, as they can burst while they're being used. A spermicide that contains the chemical Nonoxynol kills both sperms and the virus that causes AIDS; this should be used with a condom. The buying and putting on of a condom is something that can be shared. Sharing responsibility is a way of showing you care.

To sum all this up: To make sure you don't get pregnant, the pill and the IUD are the safest methods. To practise safer sex you should use a condom plus a spermicide that contains Nonoxynol. Make sure you use a brand of condom that carries the British Safety Standards kitemark on it. There's nothing to stop anyone from using both the pill and a condom plus spermicide if they're worried about both pregnancy and AIDS. (The birth control clinic you go to will advise you about this.) The responsibility for all methods can be shared in some way, whether it's helping to put on a condom or helping to remind your girlfriend to take her pill.

Legal position

It is against the law for a boy to have intercourse with a girl who is under 16 but it isn't illegal to use or get contraceptives if she's under age (see page 78). Of the four most reliable methods – the pill, the coil, the cap and the condom – only the condom and spermicides are available without medical advice. Some doctors will insist on telling a girl's parents if she asks for the pill or the coil or the cap. If she can discuss it all with her parents, well and good. But if she doesn't want them to know, she must tell her doctor this very firmly. Many doctors will then agree to go ahead and prescribe the contraceptives. Others won't, and may tell your parents or suggest another method. (The only other reliable method left is the condom.) A girl can then either decide that her boy-friend should use the condom as a way of preventing pregnancy or she can go to another doctor or clinic.

Since your National Health Service (NHS) medical card has your date of birth printed on it, there's no point in pretending that you're over 16 if you're not. None of the clinics mentioned on pages 193–4 will check up on your age, but if a girl wants the pill or coil they may ask her permission to tell her parents or family doctor. If she refuses this permission, they may go ahead and help anyway. Many doctors now recognize that any girl or boy who thinks seriously about not getting pregnant is acting responsibly.

Where to get contraception

Family doctors: can provide the following free: the pill, the coil, the cap, condoms and spermicides. Some doctors prefer to send their patients to a local family planning clinic. Because some methods can have painful or dangerous side-effects if used by girls who have had certain illnesses, a doctor who knows all about their medical history can be the best person to get advice and supplies from. If you think your doctor will tell your parents and you don't want them to know, contact one of the clinics listed on pages 193–4.

Clinics: also provide advice and supplies, usually free, to both girls and boys. Doctors or trained workers at the clinics are very helpful and friendly and can often spend more time than a family doctor with each patient, which gives them an advantage. For addresses of these centres and clinics, see pages 193–4 or look in the phone book or Yellow Pages under Family Planning.

Chemist: prescriptions for the pill can be taken to the pharmacy counter of a chemist shop. Not all chemists carry very large stocks of all brands. Condoms, spermicides and the cap can be bought over the counter (but the cap must be fitted first by a doctor or nurse to make sure you get the right size and shape).

Shops, supermarkets, surgical stores, hairdressers, etc.: you can buy condoms in lots of shops, supermarkets, etc. these days. Some surgical stores also sell the cap (you have to find out your right size from your doctor or clinic) and spermicides. Slot-machines in pubs, changing-rooms and public loos sell condoms – but always check that they carry the British Safety Standards kitemark and that the sell-by date is OK.

Live in the Republic of Ireland?

It is now possible to obtain all methods of birth control in the Republic of Ireland. If you're over 18 you can get condoms and all other non-medical contraceptives (i.e. apart from the pill and injectables) from chemists, family planning centres, VD (i.e. sexually transmitted disease) clinics or health centres, without a doctor's prescription. If you're under 18, you need a prescription to get any type of contraceptive including condoms. Contraception is not free. However, if you can't afford to pay it is still worth while having a chat with your family doctor or family planning clinic. The Irish Family Planning Association (see page 194) will advise you on methods best for you and is especially friendly.

Reliable methods

THE PILL

(combined pill,
oral contraceptive)

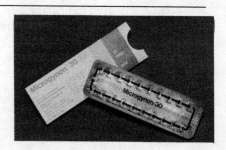

RELIABILITY

If the instructions are followed exactly, the pill is almost one hundred per cent effective.

HOW IT WORKS

The pill, which contains two chemicals, or artificial hormones (oestrogen and progestogen), is known as the combined pill. It prevents an egg from ripening and from being released from an ovary. If no egg is released, there's absolutely no chance of a girl getting pregnant. But there are several reasons why the pill is not totally one hundred per cent reliable. Sometimes a girl forgets to take her pill absolutely regularly and doesn't follow the instructions on the packet. Often a stomach upset or vomiting or diarrhoea stops the pill being absorbed by the body. It's also possible that other drugs, such as some antibiotics, prevent the pill from working properly.

DIFFERENT BRANDS

There are over thirty different brands, all a bit different and containing different amounts of the chemical hormones. Most packs have twenty-one or twenty-two pills in them: you take one each day for three weeks, stop for seven or six days when you have your period, and then start a new pack. Other brands have pills that you take every day of the year called the everyday or ED pill. All packs have instructions with them, but always ask your doctor or clinic to explain them as well. (Some manufacturers are better at making pills than writing instructions.) If a certain brand gives a girl any unwelcome effects (see below) she'll have to go back to her doctor or clinic until she finds one that suits her. Some girls never find a make of pill to suit them and have to use another method of birth control.

POINTS TO REMEMBER

Swallow a pill at the same time every day – perhaps on waking up or just before going to sleep – as this makes it easier to remember them. Follow the instructions on the pack *exactly*. For the first two weeks of taking the pill, or of taking a new brand, another method of birth control *must* be used as well. They must be swallowed every day and not just after having sex. Never lend, borrow or mix brands – because they don't work if you do. If a girl forgets to take her pill one day, she must take two the next day as soon as she remembers. If she forgets for two days on the trot, she must take all three pills as soon as she remembers, but she must then also use another birth control method until her next period starts. Being sick or having diarrhoea can get rid of the pill from the body before it's been absorbed, so another pill should be taken as soon as possible and another method of birth control must be used until the next period. Tell the doctor if you're taking any medicines as this may affect the pill.

ANNOYING SIDE-EFFECTS

While her body is getting used to the new hormone level of the pill, a girl may feel all or some of the following side-effects: tiredness, sickness (often in the morning), bleeding in between her periods, headaches, irritability, sore breasts, vaginal infections; and she may put on several pounds in weight. Sometimes a period is missed as a result of being on the pill. Any girl who misses a period and thinks she could be pregnant, should have a pregnancy test (see page 129).

Many of these side-effects go away after a month or two. If they last any longer, she must go back to her doctor or clinic and ask for another brand. If the doctor isn't very sympathetic and thinks she just has to put up with these complaints, the best plan is to go to another doctor or clinic.

SERIOUS SIDE-EFFECTS

It's possible that some people exaggerate the dangers of the pill because they don't like the thought of women being able to control the number of babies they have so easily and efficiently – there are still a surprising number of people around who think that you should only have sex if you plan to have a baby! But on the other hand, not nearly enough research has been done on the pill for us to know about all the possible dangers and side-effects. The medical experts now think that anyone taking it for four years at a time should give it a rest for a few months before going back on it. No woman over 40 should take the pill and those over 30 should think very seriously about the possible side-effects – especially if they've been on the pill for some years. Don't take the pill if you smoke more than one or two cigarettes a day as it could increase the chances of heart disease.

You should tell your doctor if you have suffered from any of the following complaints and diseases – or if there is a history of them in your family: varicose veins, blood clotting, strokes, heart disease of any kind, cancer of the breast or internal sex organs, hepatitis, jaundice or any liver disease, diabetes, kidney disease, high blood pressure, sickle-cell anaemia or trait (black girls planning to go on the pill should have a test for this disease), epilepsy, asthma, migraine headaches, breast tumours, fibroids in the womb, depression, cystic fibrosis. There may be a connection between the pill and cancer. Sufferers from these complaints and women who are breastfeeding may be warned against taking the pill.

Anything unusual that you think might be a result of taking the pill that lasts for more than about two months *must* be reported to the doctor or clinic.

You may find that taking the pill makes you lose all sexual desire. In this case, the pill is definitely not the best method of birth control for you.

DISADVANTAGES

Most of the possible disadvantages have been described under the above section on side-effects. For a girl who doesn't want her parents to know she's on the pill, hiding the packet may prove a problem. It's *not* a good idea to take them out of their packet and put them in a bottle as this makes it almost impossible to remember whether they've been taken each day. Many women dislike taking artificial hormones and chemicals because so little is known about the possible consequences.

ADVANTAGES

As long as the instructions are followed exactly the pill gives complete protection against unwanted pregnancies. Many women find that once they're on the pill all their worries and fears about getting pregnant disappear and their sex life improves enormously. The pill often makes women feel much better just before their periods and it usually makes periods much shorter and less painful. It may clear up a spotty complexion.

THE MINI-PILL

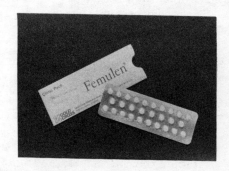

RELIABILITY

Out of every hundred women who take the mini-pill for a year, about two get pregnant.

HOW IT WORKS

Many doctors believed in the past that some of the side-effects of the ordinary pill were caused by oestrogen, one of the two artificial hormones. The mini-pill has only one of these hormones (progestogen) and was introduced to solve these problems, although now it's thought that it is in fact progestogen which is responsible for the side-effects. This particular hormone makes the mucus inside the neck of the womb much thicker than usual and so sperms find it impossible to get through and into the womb and fallopian tubes.

POINTS TO REMEMBER

The mini-pill has to be swallowed every single day of the year. It *must* be taken absolutely regularly and at exactly the same time each day. If it's taken even a few hours later than usual on one day, it may not prevent pregnancy.

DISADVANTAGES

It's not as reliable as the combined pill and even less is known about the possible long-term side-effects. It often causes heavy and irregular periods for the first few months. Many women find it almost impossible to take at the same time every day because they don't lead clockwork lives.

ADVANTAGES

It's a better pill for girls who are overweight or who have a personal or family medical history of blood clotting, diabetes, asthma, epilepsy, migraine or liver disease.

THE MORNING-AFTER (POST-COITAL) PILL

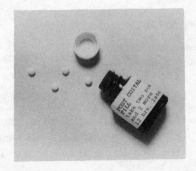

RELIABILITY

If taken no later than three days after unprotected sex this usually prevents pregnancy. The sooner you take these pills the more effective they are.

HOW IT WORKS

A doctor will prescribe two special doses of special pills (ordinary contraceptive pills don't work) that have to be taken twelve hours apart. This alters the hormone balance in your body and prevents pregnancy.

DISADVANTAGES

You may feel and actually be sick. If you are sick, go back to the doctor or clinic immediately. This method of birth control is not suitable for all girls and women – only a doctor can advise you. And it's only an emergency method – you can't use it every time you have sex.

THE COIL
(Intrauterine device,
IUD, loop)

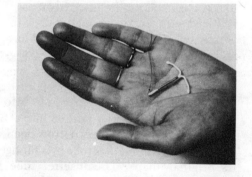

RELIABILITY

Out of every hundred women who use the coil for a year, about two get pregnant.

HOW IT WORKS

Intrauterine means 'inside the uterus', which is where the coil is fitted. They're small, flat, flexible metal or plastic devices which only a properly trained person can fit into the womb. They come in various shapes. They all have a couple of threads attached to the end.

No one is quite sure how the coil works. It touches the womb in several places and seems to prevent a fertilized egg from attaching itself to the sides of the womb. It's also thought that it makes the egg travel down the fallopian tube much faster than usual so that the lining of the womb just isn't ready to accept a fertilized egg when it has arrived there. It is possible that the coil irritates the womb lining and large white blood cells are then produced in the womb which destroy the egg and sperms.

INSERTING THE COIL

Fitting a coil into the womb is quite simple but it has to be done by someone who is specially trained. Not all family doctors are trained to do it, so it may be better and safer to go to one of the clinics mentioned on pages 193–4. Anyone can be fitted with a coil although it used to be thought that only women who have had babies could have one. (Some doctors and clinics won't give the coil to a girl who hasn't had a baby.)

Every coil, whatever its shape, is flexible enough to be pressed into a straight line and put into a very narrow tube. This tube is then gently pushed into the vagina, and up into the womb through the very narrow opening in the cervix. The coil is pushed out of this tube by a plunger and it goes back to its original shape. The inserter tube is then pulled out, leaving the coil in the womb with its threads hanging down through the cervix into the very top of the vagina.

The whole process is very quick – less than half a minute or so. It can hurt, sometimes quite a lot, especially if the girl is very tense. But some women hardly feel a thing.

DISADVANTAGES

The womb isn't used to having anything solid in it and so it often tries to push the coil out. This can cause cramp pains and bleeding – especially just after it's been inserted. Medicines normally taken for period pains and a hot water bottle can make a girl feel more comfortable.

You have to go to the doctor or clinic to have the coil removed but sometimes the coil gets pushed out of its own accord. Some girls find it stays in the second or third time, others find that they can never keep one in. Because it's so easy for a coil to be pushed out and flushed away unnoticed, a girl must check that it's still there once a week. The best way to do this is in the bath or squatting down, pushing a finger or two up inside the vagina and feeling for the little threads. If the threads aren't there or the coil itself can be felt pushing its way out, a visit to the doctor or clinic is called for. In the meantime another birth control method must be used.

A coil can cause more serious complications. It's been noticed that many women with coils develop severe infections in their internal sex organs. Very rarely, it can pierce the wall of the womb. Any severe pain or bleeding should be reported to the doctor immediately. So should continued pain of any kind.

A girl with a coil who misses a period or becomes pregnant should also immediately visit her doctor. It can cause complications during pregnancy, although not always, but a doctor will have to make sure.

ADVANTAGES

The coil can be put in and forgotten – apart from the girl's own weekly check. Most coils can be left in for four years. It's one of the few birth control methods that's completely separate from sex – once it's in you don't have to think about birth control again. It's almost as safe as the pill but doesn't involve taking chemicals or produce any of their side-effects.

THE MORNING-AFTER COIL

RELIABILITY

If used no more than five days after unprotected sex this is a very reliable method of birth control. The sooner you get one fitted, the more reliable it is.

HOW IT WORKS

A doctor will fit a coil into your womb and this should prevent any fertilized egg from becoming implanted.

DISADVANTAGES

The coil isn't suitable for all girls and women. The disadvantages of the coil mentioned above all apply.

THE CONDOM

(johnny, french letter, noddy, rubber, Durex, Mates, sheath, safe, preventative, prophylactic, etc.)

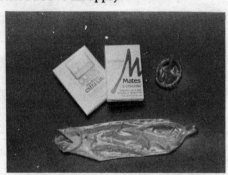

RELIABILITY

Out of every hundred couples using the condom for a year, about four women become pregnant. It's even more reliable when used with a spermicide as well (see page 120).

HOW IT WORKS

A condom is made of very thin rubber and fits on to an erect penis before intercourse. When the boy ejaculates, his semen and sperms stay inside the condom. This means that the sperms don't get into the vagina and can't swim up into the womb.

It has to be put on very carefully, holding the closed end firmly between the fingers and thumb while it's being rolled

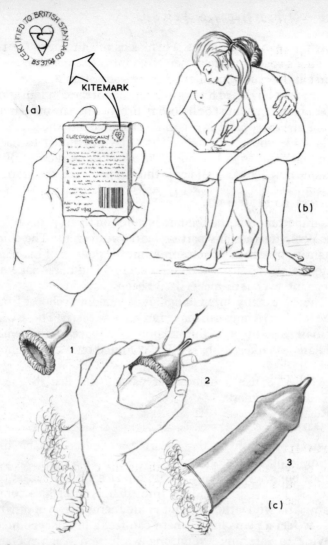

(a)

CERTIFIED TO BRITISH STANDARD

BS3704

KITEMARK

ELECTRONICALLY TESTED

(b)

1

2

3

(c)

Helping each other to put on a condom is just one of the ways in which a couple can share fun and the responsibility of birth control.

1. A rolled-up condom with a teat looks like this when it is taken out of its package.
2. Condoms with teats are a lot less likely to burst than those without. One of you has to squeeze the teat as you're putting it on to prevent any air getting trapped in the end of the condom.

down over the erect penis. This keeps the air out of the tip, leaving a space for the semen to go into. The condom could burst at the crucial moment if there's any air in it.

After the boy's had his orgasm, the rim of the condom at the base of his penis must be held very firmly while he pulls it out of the girl's vagina. If any sperms get spilled into the vagina at this stage you might as well not have bothered to use a condom at all. A girl should always use some sperm-killing chemical in her vagina, in case this happens (see page 120).

POINTS TO REMEMBER

It's important that the condom is rolled on to the penis before the penis touches any part of a girl's sex organs. The small quantity of semen which sometimes leaks out of his penis before a boy comes can contain sperms and may make her pregnant, even if the penis hasn't been inside her.

There are many different brands of condom to choose from. The lubricated ones can make intercourse easier. Those with a small bag, or teat, at the end provide a space for the semen and are less likely to burst. The coloured ones can be more fun.

ALWAYS use a brand that carries the British Safety Standards kitemark.

DISADVANTAGES

Many boys complain that wearing a condom is a bit like trying to play the guitar with gloves on. This is an exaggeration, but they do tend to cut down a bit on sensation. Because he has to withdraw immediately after he's come, many girls who either haven't come themselves yet or who like to feel a penis inside them can feel a bit disappointed. Having to interrupt everything while you reach for and unwrap a condom can cause some problems – especially if he finds his penis shrinks at this stage.

ADVANTAGES

They're easy to buy and simple to use. Many couples find the whole business of putting them on – and it's something you can do together – a real turn-on. If you've never used one before and you think you might be a bit shy with your partner, a boy might practise – and perhaps enjoy – using a condom on his own when he masturbates. Condoms help to prevent the spread of sexually transmitted diseases. Doctors who are worried by the number of young girls who get tendencies towards cancer of the cervix recommend the condom.

The condom is an absolute must for safer sex. Sexually transmitted diseases can't get past the barrier of a condom. But because they can burst they must always be used with a spermicide which kills the virus that causes AIDS as well as sperms (see page 120).

Warning: there are mini-condoms that cover only the tip of the penis called 'Grecian tips' or 'American tips'. These are totally useless – DON'T use them.

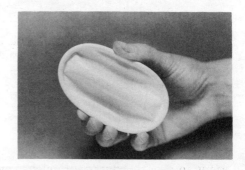

THE CAP
(diaphragm, dutch cap)

RELIABILITY

Out of every hundred women using the cap with a sperm-killing chemical for a year, about four get pregnant.

HOW IT WORKS

A cap looks a bit like a small shallow bowl. The dome is made of thin rubber and the thicker rim is made of flexible wire covered in rubber. There are some smaller plastic types (called cervical caps) for girls who are allergic to rubber.

They fit inside the vagina and close off the entrance to the womb so that sperms all stay in the vagina. If any do manage

1. Apply
   spermicide
   inside and
   outside the cap.

2. Take up a
   comfortable
   position.

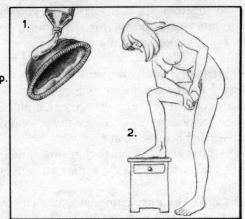

3. Squeeze the
   cap and put it
   in the vagina.
   (The dome
   should be facing
   forwards.)

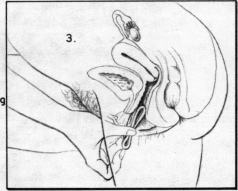

4. The cap is in
   the correct
   position.
   A finger checks
   that it is
   covering the
   cervix.

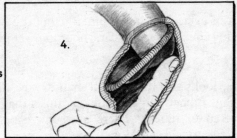

to wriggle past they're killed by the spermicide, which must be used with a cap.

FITTING

No two girls have exactly the same size or shape of vagina so everyone has to be fitted individually by her doctor or clinic. She'll be given an internal examination which involves lying on her back with her legs spread apart. The doctor or nurse will gently feel inside her vagina with their fingers and show her how to put the cap in. Don't leave the clinic or doctor until you've tried putting it in yourself and can do it easily. After a bit of practice they're very easy to use.

HOW TO USE

A cap has to be put in place no more than three hours before intercourse. A splurge of spermicide cream or jelly (about a teaspoonful) must be smeared on each side of the dome, and some more spread all the way round the rim. The cap is then squeezed between the fingers and thumb into a cigar shape and pushed up into the vagina so that the cervix is completely covered. A girl must then check if it's properly in place with her finger. The cap must cover the cervix. This feels like a small knob right up inside the vagina. When the cap's in place, this knob can be felt behind the centre of the cap.

If you have intercourse more than three hours after putting the cap in, don't remove it but squeeze some more spermicide up your vagina. (Spermicides come with special applicators just for this purpose.) Don't take it out for at least six hours, preferably eight hours, after intercourse to make sure that all the sperms are killed, and don't leave it in for more than twenty-four hours. It's usually easier to take it out by crouching or lifting one leg up.

POINTS TO REMEMBER

Never borrow or lend your cap – your friend isn't necessarily going to be the same size or shape. Go for another fitting if you put on or lose more than half a stone in weight. If you get fitted for a cap before you've ever had intercourse you must go for another fitting afterwards – you may need another size.

After use, the cap must be washed gently in warm water and mild soap, rinsed and then dried *very* thoroughly. Inspect for defects or holes by holding it up to the light. If it gets bent out of shape, just bend the rim gently back to its circular shape.

A cap can't disappear up inside or get stuck in the vagina. The only way out for anything as big as a cap is the way it went in.

DISADVANTAGES

Having to think about putting in a cap before sex can be a bit of a drawback. It is possible for a cap to slip or get pushed out of place during intercourse, which is why they should ALWAYS be used with a spermicide. Sometimes the cap can be felt by the tip of the penis – although this shouldn't happen if it's properly in place. It occasionally feels a bit uncomfortable to take the cap out.

ADVANTAGES

If used properly, looked after carefully (beware of long finger-nails) and always used with a spermicide, caps are a reliable method of birth control. Many women like to feel that they're not swallowing chemicals or placing some metal or plastic object permanently into their wombs and yet are still controlling for themselves whether or not they get pregnant. Caps are also a good way of temporarily holding back the flow if you have sex during a period. Some doctors believe that the cap, like the condom, may help prevent a tendency to cancer of the cervix.

Spermicides with the chemical Nonoxynol kill both sperms and the virus that can cause AIDS. Check on the packet or ask the chemist.

SPERMICIDES

RELIABILITY

NOT reliable on their own. MUST be used with condom or cap.

HOW THEY WORK

There are three main types of chemical contraceptives that kill sperms: jellies and creams, tablets (called pessaries) that go into the vagina, and aerosol foams. The foams both kill sperms and make a thick barrier so that sperms can't swim into the womb. The jellies and creams come with a plunger-type applicator that you push into your vagina.

DISADVANTAGES

Use only the brands recommended by the doctor or clinic – some brands can make caps and condoms perish and can cause soreness if either girl or boy is allergic to the chemical. After sex the spermicides leak out which can be rather messy, but the girl shouldn't have a bath until about six hours after because water and soap can get inside and dilute or affect the spermicide. Couples who enjoy each other's natural tastes and smells find that spermicides don't always taste too good, but they're not poisonous.

Warning: Ignore all claims made by manufacturers that spermicides can be used on their own – they can't. One particular brand, called 'C-Film' (advertised as the first his-and-hers contraceptive), which supposedly fits over the tip of the penis or can be put inside the vagina, should NOT be used as a contraceptive.

ADVANTAGES

No prescription is needed – you can buy them at any chemist – although they're quite expensive and you can get them free from the clinic. Some brands help prevent the spread of sexually transmitted diseases.

Because of the possibility of catching the virus that causes AIDS, ALWAYS use a brand that contains the chemical Nonoxynol. The chemist will help you get the right sort. Nonoxynol kills both sperms and the virus on contact.

INJECTABLES
(the jab, the jag)

RELIABILITY

For every hundred women using it for one year, virtually none will get pregnant.

HOW IT WORKS

A doctor injects a hormone, usually into your arm, during the first five days of your period. There are two different sorts: one injection of Depo-Provera lasts for twelve weeks; one injection of Noristerat lasts for eight weeks. This hormone is very similar to the hormone progestogen used in the mini-pill.

DISADVANTAGES

They are generally only given to girls and women who really can't use any other method of birth control – either because they can't for medical reasons or because they never remember to use another method. Few girls or young women are given injectables. The side-effects are very similar to those of the mini-pill. Periods may become lighter and disappear, or there may be some light bleeding all the time. If it doesn't suit you, you have to wait and live with the side-effects for eight to twelve weeks, depending on which sort you've been given. Some women remain infertile for a long time after they've been injected. Research is still being carried out on the possible links between injectables and cervical cancer.

STERILIZATION

All the birth control methods described above can be reversed. That's to say anyone who decides they do want a baby can simply stop using whatever method it is that they've been using. Sterilization is not reversible. Although some women and men who have been sterilized and then changed their minds have had operations to reverse the original one, there's no guarantee that this can be done.

For women, sterilization involves an operation either to tie off or block both fallopian tubes or burn the ends of the tubes so that no egg ever reaches the womb.

For men, an operation called a vasectomy is done, tying off or blocking the tubes which carry the sperm to the seminal fluid. He can still have a perfectly normal orgasm and ejaculation, but there aren't any sperms in the semen.

Anyone wanting to be sterilized must be absolutely sure that they won't want children in the future. Doctors dislike doing these operations on anyone who is under 30, who is unmarried or hasn't had at least one child.

The operation used to be done only if it was thought that the mother might have diseased babies. There have been cases of parents or guardians arranging for young girls to be sterilized for this reason, but this is very rare.

Unreliable methods

The following methods should not be used unless you don't mind if you have a baby.

NATURAL METHODS

RELIABILITY

Out of every hundred couples who use these methods, thirty or more will get pregnant.

HOW THEY'RE SUPPOSED TO WORK

Many girls and boys have a vague idea that there are certain times of the month when it's 'safe' to have sex and she won't get pregnant. Depending on what they've heard, some think it's safe to have sex during a girl's period, others think it's safe to have it just before or just after. The truth is that no one can ever be certain of when it is or isn't absolutely 'safe'. A girl may ovulate at any time, even though she thinks she knows she's absolutely regular.

There are three natural methods. The temperature method means taking your temperature every day and keeping a chart. After ovulation her temperature rises a little bit. Certain days before and after this temperature rise are the one of greatest risk. The Billings or mucus method is used by many couples in the Republic of Ireland. The woman or girl has to feel the mucus or secretions in her vagina every day to find out the time when she is unlikely to get pregnant. The calendar method involves keeping a check on her menstrual cycle for six months to a year to try to work out when the 'safest' time might be.

DISADVANTAGES

Although there are clearly no health risks to any of these methods, they are very complicated – you'll need some help from a doctor to show you how to do any of them – and none of these methods are a good idea for any couple who definitely don't want to have a baby. Clearly, these methods won't protect either partner from AIDS or any other sexually transmitted disease.

WITHDRAWAL
(coitus interruptus, pulling out in time, being careful)

RELIABILITY

Out of every hundred couples using this method for a year, about seventeen get pregnant.

HOW IT'S SUPPOSED TO WORK

Just before he has his orgasm, the boy has to pull his penis out of the vagina and make sure that no sperms get anywhere near her vagina.

DISADVANTAGES

This 'method' accounts for a high number of unwanted babies and teenage pregnancies. Sperms can leak from the penis before a boy ejaculates – and it only takes one particularly hardy sperm to make a girl pregnant. It's also possible for AIDS and other sexually transmitted diseases to be passed on this way. It can be very difficult for a boy to withdraw in time, however experienced he is.

It can also limit the possible positions in which you can have sex – it is very difficult for a couple to suddenly spring apart at just the right time if she is sitting on top of him. Withdrawing suddenly can spoil his orgasm and can also spoil sex for her. It's very doubtful that she will ever be able to feel really satisfied if this 'method' is used.

HOLDING BACK
(coitus reservatus)

RELIABILITY

NOT reliable.

HOW IT'S SUPPOSED TO WORK

According to the rule of this 'method', once the penis has entered the vagina, you both have to lie absolutely still and wait for the penis to go limp and little. And that's it! The boy then pulls out his penis without either of you having an orgasm.

DISADVANTAGES

As with withdrawing, it's very possible for some sperms to leak out of the penis before the boy has an orgasm. The amount of self-control needed is enormous. It's difficult to imagine how anyone could possibly enjoy sex by this method.

DOUCHE
(pronounced 'doosh')

RELIABILITY
NOT reliable – possibly *increases* the chances of pregnancy.

HOW IT'S SUPPOSED TO WORK
A douche (which is the French word for a shower) is a rubber bulb which is filled with a special chemical. It has a long rubber tube attached which is pushed into the vagina. By squeezing the bulb, the solution rushes into the vagina and washes it out. Immediately after she's had intercourse a girl is supposed to run into the bathroom and use her douche. The big problem with this as a birth control method is that sperms swim into the womb a whole lot quicker than anyone can run to the bathroom. And instead of killing sperms and washing them out, the pressure of the solution may actually help push sperms *into* the womb.

Warning: some doctors recommend a douche to cure certain vaginal infections – other doctors believe that it's possible to damage a girl's internal sex organs in this way. Should only ever be used under close medical supervision.

SPONGE
('Today' sponge)

RELIABILITY
Out of every hundred women using the sponge for a year, about twenty-five will get pregnant.

HOW IT'S SUPPOSED TO WORK
The 'Today' contraceptive sponge is mushroom-shaped with a loop attached and about the size of a marshmallow. It's made of soft polyurethane and is impregnated with a strong spermicide. You buy it, without prescription, from the chemist. After moistening it with tap water (to start the release of

the spermicide) you push it high up into the vagina so that it covers the neck of the womb. It can be put in from a few seconds to twenty-four hours before sex. Leave it in for at least six hours after love-making. Take it out by pulling on its loop. You then throw it away.

ADVANTAGES

Only of value as a back-up for other methods such as the condom.

DISADVANTAGES

Because it's not at all effective at preventing you from getting pregnant, the sponge is not suitable for highly fertile young women not ready for pregnancy. It shouldn't be used by girls or women of any age who *must not* get pregnant.

CHAPTER NINE

Pregnancy

Even before you can possibly tell you might be pregnant, if you had sex without using any birth control or if the condom you were using burst, there are two morning-after methods which will prevent an unplanned pregnancy. You have to act quickly because the longer you leave it the less likely they are to work. See 'The morning-after pill' on page 110 and 'The morning-after coil' on page 114. These are only emergency methods of birth control. You can't use them every time you have intercourse.

How to tell

It's not always easy for a girl to tell if she's pregnant. As soon as the egg has been fertilized by a sperm, hormones are produced which prevent any more eggs from ripening and she won't have any more periods until the pregnancy is ended. So missing a period may be the first sign of pregnancy. But few girls ever know exactly when to expect their periods – they're often very irregular. A late period or missing out on one altogether can also be because a girl's hormones haven't yet become properly balanced or simply the result of dieting, over-tiredness, a change in routine or an emotional upset. Worrying about being pregnant can also make her miss a period. It's a good idea for a girl to keep a record of when she has her periods so she'll have some idea of whether her period is late or how late it is. There can be several other signs of pregnancy. Morning sickness – either feeling or being sick – is common during the first three months of a pregnancy. Her breasts may swell slightly and feel a bit sore.

If you haven't had sex since your last period, you're probably not pregnant. But, occasionally, you can get a false period during early pregnancy. Some light bleeding lasting maybe only a day or two, plus some other signs like tiredness, sickness and wanting to pee very often, probably means that you are pregnant.

The only way to find out is to have a pregnancy test. No test can be accurate until a few days after your period is late. This is why it's such a good idea to keep a note of when you expect your periods if you're having a sexual relationship. Many girls waste valuable time, just hoping that their period will come. The sooner you find out the sooner you'll be able to get the necessary advice. Speed is essential if you think you may want an abortion. In any case, you'll need as much time as possible to think about what you want to do if you are pregnant.

Despite all the rumours, there are no pills or medicines that a doctor will automatically prescribe or that you can buy which will bring on your period if you are pregnant after the first few days (see page 111). There are pills that doctors can prescribe which bring on a period in a girl who isn't pregnant, but few doctors like prescribing these for a young girl.

Some girls think they can bring on a period by taking a hot bath, jumping down flights of stairs or taking a bike ride over a bumpy field. They're probably more than half hoping that if they *are* pregnant this will give them a miscarriage (an accidental spontaneous abortion). But none of these or any other methods work. If they did, all women would be able to have their periods whenever they wanted, or every time they fell over!

Pregnancy testing

You can either buy a do-it-yourself testing kit from the chemist or go to your doctor, to a family planning clinic or to a pregnancy advisory clinic (for addresses, see pages 193–4). Some brands of the do-it-yourself kits are fairly reliable just a few days after your period is late. With others you have to wait until two weeks after your period was due. All you need for the test is a sample of some early-morning pee.

If the result is positive (meaning that you are pregnant), then you almost certainly are. A negative result (suggesting that you're not pregnant) may be wrong. If you get a negative result and your period still hasn't come, do another test four or five days later.

Doctors and family planning or pregnancy advisory clinics may be able to do the test for you while you wait. Take along a sample of your early-morning pee in a small clean bottle or jar with an airtight lid on it. An old pill bottle or small herb jar is ideal. Wash it out first with some water that you've boiled.

Once you've missed two periods, a doctor will be able to tell if you're pregnant by giving an internal examination. For this you undress from the waist down and lie on your back with your legs spread apart. The doctor will wear a lubricated glove to feel inside your vagina. Go with your boyfriend or a friend if you can't face this on your own. The doctors in the clinics won't mind.

If you're not pregnant

The only way to make sure you don't have to go through all that worry and hassle again is to make sure that you use a really reliable method of birth control (see page 99).

If you were using an effective contraceptive, go back and read the chapter again to check whether you've been using it properly.

If you are pregnant

A girl who is pregnant but didn't plan to be can have an abortion or stay pregnant. If she has the child she can choose to keep it or arrange to have it adopted or fostered. If you're under 16 you can't get married (see page 146). Some girls plan to keep their baby and marry the father as soon as they're old enough. For anyone under 16 the chances are that the decision will be taken for them. But it may not be the right decision. Try to work out in your own mind what you want and why. If your parents try to persuade you to have your baby and get it adopted, but you want an abortion, it won't be easy to do what you want to do. But it may be possible.

If you are pregnant and you think you may have the virus that causes AIDS, you may want to think about having a test to check this out. This test is called the HIV (Human Immunodeficiency Virus) antibody test. It can't tell you if you have AIDS itself, but it can tell you if you have the virus that causes AIDS in your bloodstream. The reason for having this test if you're pregnant is as follows: people can have this HIV virus and not be aware of it for several years. Not everyone with the HIV virus automatically gets the full AIDS illness. But a pregnant woman with the HIV virus is far more likely to develop AIDS. And a baby born to a woman with this virus could be born infected and become ill with AIDS itself. You can have this test done by your family doctor, or it can be arranged through an ante-natal clinic, or you can go to a special clinic which deals with sexually transmitted diseases (for the address of your nearest special clinic see page 193). If you do have this virus, the result is called HIV antibody positive. If you don't, it's called HIV antibody negative. Knowing whether or not you have the HIV virus may affect your decision about whether or not to have an abortion. (For more about this test, see page 165.)

First reactions

Doubtless if you didn't intend getting pregnant your first reaction will be one of panic. This doesn't help, but it's natural to think that your whole life, career and family will be in ruins. In fact, nothing need be ruined, although this won't be easy to imagine at the time.

Some girls who can't face the family reaction decide just to run away from home. This is a very bad idea. With nowhere to go or stay, worse things than being pregnant can happen to you, especially if you're under 16. The best that can happen is that you'll be found and brought back home – probably by the police. By this time you'll be in trouble with your parents and the police.

Do not try to have a 'do-it-yourself' abortion. There are no pills you can get to give yourself and end your pregnancy. Boiling hot baths, drinking a bottle of gin or falling downstairs only produce third-degree burns, big hangovers or broken necks. If any of these methods worked there would be no unwanted babies in the world. The two most dangerous things a girl can do are to try to abort herself or go to an illegal 'back street' abortionist. No one, not even a qualified doctor or nurse, can do an abortion legally or safely unless it's been arranged through the proper organizations (see page 193). You can end up killing yourself or being killed.

Some girls think about committing suicide. A few try it. But being pregnant is not the end of the world – you do have some choice and there are people to help you.

With some careful thought and planning it's possible to find the right solution for you. And within a few weeks or months the nightmare of an unwanted pregnancy can all be over. The first thing to realize is that you can't go through it all alone.

Who to tell

Almost certainly a girl is going to have to tell her parents in the end, especially if she's under 16. But it may help to talk to someone else first.

BOYFRIEND

The most natural person to tell is the boy involved, if you know who it is. Boys can react in many different ways. He may turn out to be the most kind and helpful friend in the world. Or he may turn out nasty and not want to know. Or he may panic more than the girl. If she is under 16, he has broken the law (see page 78). So when he hears that his girlfriend is pregnant, apart from being scared and worried, he may also have a vivid picture of himself in the arms of the law. The boy has no rights over you or the baby, however much he might like to be a father.

FRIEND

A friend – especially one who has been through all this herself – can be a great help. An older friend, neighbour or relative may help tell your parents. But however close or good your friend might be, she or he won't necessarily know what to do any more than you do.

TEACHER

There are some teachers who will do little more than throw up their hands in horror. But there are many who will be kind and helpful. The chances are that your form teacher will have a pretty good idea of what's up in any case. A sympathetic teacher can be a very good ally if you're expecting trouble at home. One of your parents' worries will be about your education. Your teacher should be able to help you with this problem.

PERSONNEL OFFICER

Some factories and firms employ personnel staff to help their workers with problems such as this. You may want extra time off from work to get all the medical advice you'll need and the personnel officer should be able to help arrange this.

PROFESSIONAL ADVICE

If a girl hasn't visited her doctor she'll have to quite soon. She'll need to get the medical attention that every pregnant woman needs, or to discuss the possibility of getting an abortion. An abortion has to be done quickly because after three months it is both dangerous and nearly impossible to get one. And it can take time to arrange.

There are various organizations a girl can go to for concrete help and advice. The law requires that the parents of a girl under 16 sign the consent form for an abortion operation. If you don't want your parents to know, say so and explain why. They'll still give you advice and help (including help on how to tell your parents). Most large towns have at least one of the organizations or clinics mentioned on pages 193–4 you can go to. Phone them first to see if you need an appointment or have to pay a fee. Their advice is only 'professional' in the sense that it will be good and accurate, not bossy. They are informal and often very friendly.

PARENTS

Your parents may be the best people in the world to tell once you've found the courage – or they may be the worst. But, in either case, if you live at home or are under 16 they'll have to be told. The chances are that their first reaction will be the same as yours – panic. If they didn't know you were having a sexual relationship they may be very shocked. They might feel angry, hurt, disgraced, ashamed, or a mixture of all these things.

Their reactions can range from worrying about how your education will be affected to what the neighbours will think. If you have younger sisters and brothers they'll probably worry about whether they should be told. It's more than likely that a lot of things will get said which will later be regretted.

Parents can be surprising. Many will give you a lot of support. Some who for years have been warning their daughter that she'll get thrown out of the house if she ever gets pregnant turn out to be really kind and realistic. But they may not know what to do. If you have made the effort to contact an organization which can help, your parents may realize that you're not as irresponsible as they thought. After all, for many girls getting pregnant is simply an accident.

It will help if you can try to understand how they feel and why. Hopefully they'll try to understand how you feel as well. One thing's certain: endless rows and discussions about how and why you got pregnant won't help at all. A decision on what to do has to be made – and soon.

CHAPTER TEN

Abortion

An abortion means that a doctor ends, or terminates, a pregnancy. It's a very controversial subject. There are those who campaign to make abortion free and available to every woman 'on demand' so that every child is a wanted child. Others are very much opposed to abortion and want to make it impossible or very much harder to get than it already is.

Those who are against abortion argue on religious and humane grounds that an unborn child, called a foetus (pronounced fee-tuss), has as much right to live as a born child. They point out that having an abortion can cause mental and physical complications for the pregnant woman. They say that unwanted babies give a lot of happiness to childless couples wanting to adopt. Some believe that many women are pressured into having an abortion because society does not make it easy for a single woman to keep her child.

Those in favour of abortion being available (the pro-choice lobby) don't think it makes sense to talk of a foetus as a child until it's actually been born or until the time after it was conceived when it might survive if it was born early. They point out that no method of birth control is one hundred per cent safe and that it's unfair to make women suffer just because their contraceptive failed. Unwanted and unplanned children can result in misery, poverty, battered babies, unhappy people or broken families.

The mental and physical complications which can follow from having a baby and then giving it away can be far greater than any complications which may result from having an abortion. Many women feel that they should have the right to control their own bodies and the number of children they have and that this should not be left up to (mostly male) scientists and politicians. They argue that if abortion is illegal it will mean that, once again, rich women will be able to get safe abortions but women without the money will be forced to have dangerous, back street abortions.

If you are thinking about having an abortion you'll probably be weighing up the arguments for and against – but you'll also be thinking of your own particular situation. Before you take your decision talk it over with your doctor or a counsellor at one of the pregnancy advisory services mentioned on pages 193–4.

How safe?

Whatever your feelings are it's important to get some facts straight. Any operation involves some risk, and an abortion is no exception. The sooner you have your abortion the safer it is. But it is actually safer to have an abortion than it is to be pregnant and have a baby.

There are other possible complications both in having an abortion and in being pregnant. An abortion can cause an infected or damaged womb. Or it may cause your cervix to become so stretched that it makes it difficult to have a baby in the future. It can cause such heavy bleeding that a blood transfusion will be needed.

But these things can also happen to women who continue in their pregnancy, either by having a miscarriage (an accidental, spontaneous abortion), or while giving birth.

How to get an abortion

According to the law you can get a legal abortion provided two doctors sign a form agreeing that one or more of the following things is true:

—To continue being pregnant would mean a greater risk to your life than to have an abortion.

—To continue being pregnant would mean a greater risk to your physical or mental health than to have an abortion.

—To continue being pregnant would involve a greater risk to the physical or mental health of any other children in your family than to have an abortion.

—There is reasonable suspicion that the child will be born seriously mentally or physically handicapped.

—If the pregnant girl or woman has the HIV virus that can cause AIDS, or AIDS itself, this is usually accepted as a good enough reason for an abortion.

IF YOU ARE UNDER 16

You will need the written consent of your parents, guardians or your social worker if you are in care. The majority of girls under 16 in most areas get an abortion free on the National Health Service. No NHS doctor would agree to do an abortion without getting this written consent. If you go to one of the private charitable pregnancy advisory services listed on pages 193–4 they will also need your parents' written permission, but they are very sympathetic to the problems that many young girls have. Explain to the counsellor exactly what your personal situation and problem is.

GETTING A FREE ABORTION ON THE NATIONAL HEALTH SERVICE

Go to your own doctor, and explain why you want an abortion. You'll be given an internal examination. Some doctors don't approve of abortion and will either refuse to sign the form or refuse to let you have it on the NHS. If you can afford to pay, your doctor may take the view that you should have it done privately to make room in hospital for a woman who can't afford an abortion. If your doctor does not agree to an abortion, the best plan is to go to a doctor at a non-profit-making pregnancy advisory service centre.

If your doctor agrees, she or he will arrange for you to see a gynaecologist who is a specialist in these matters, at a hospital. When you see the gynaecologist, explain to her or him why you want an abortion. You will be given an internal examination. You may be sent to a psychiatrist if the specialist wants to find out how your pregnancy is affecting your mental state. If the specialist agrees to an abortion you will be told when you can go into hospital. In the hospital you may find yourself in a ward with other women happily expecting babies and women who are trying to find out why they can't have babies at all; this can be very upsetting for everyone. Make sure you take plenty of magazines or books to try to take your mind off it all when you need to.

Arranging for an abortion is seldom just as easy as this. In some towns and areas it can be easier than in others, depending on how long the waiting list is for beds at hospitals and how sympathetic the health authority or individual doctors are. But if your doctors seem to be delaying, don't delay yourself. If you get to be ten weeks pregnant (i.e. it is ten weeks since your last period) and you have no immediate date fixed for a hospital bed, go to one of the pregnancy advisory services to try and arrange for a private abortion.

PRIVATE OR CHARITABLE ABORTION SERVICES

The organizations listed on pages 193–4 all provide non-profit-making advisory services. They charge as little as possible but you should expect to pay up to £200. The later you leave it the more expensive it is. They can sometimes arrange a free NHS abortion even if you've already been refused one. They may be able to give you financial help such as an interest-free loan. If you belong to one of the private patient schemes like British United Provident Association (BUPA) or Private Patients Plus (PPP) you should be able to claim back the money.

Check on the phone beforehand whether you need an appointment. There's often a long queue. You'll have a talk with a counsellor and then be given an appointment to see a doctor. If the doctor agrees, you'll be booked into a clinic or nursing home which is specially licensed by the government to give abortions. Find out who and when you have to pay from the advisory service. You may not be allowed visitors, but the atmosphere is usually very friendly and nearly everyone is there for the same reason.

COMMERCIAL ABORTION SERVICES

There are a number of commercial pregnancy advisory services which give abortions at high prices in order to make a profit. They send women to private gynaecologists and private clinics, who also charge high fees. All clinics have to be licensed and the government occasionally removes the licence from a clinic or nursing home that doesn't come up to standard. If you are not sure if your advisory service or clinic is as cheap as it could be, or might not be properly licensed, phone the British Pregnancy Advisory Service to check (page 193).

LIVE IN NORTHERN IRELAND?

Abortion is not legal in Northern Ireland and you can usually only get your pregnancy terminated for strictly medical reasons. Ulster Pregnancy Advisory Association Ltd (address, page 195) provides a counselling service and can then refer you to the British Pregnancy Advisory Service clinic in Liverpool. Many women go to England for the operation. If you decide to go to England, phone one of the charitable advisory services on pages 193–4 to get a definite appointment before you leave. They won't be able to guarantee an abortion until they've seen you, but they'll probably make a provisional booking at a clinic or nursing home within a day or two of your first appointment so that you won't have to stay away from home too long.

LIVE IN THE REPUBLIC OF IRELAND?

Abortion is illegal in the Republic of Ireland, but there is an informal network of agencies which can arrange abortions in

England. If you can't get in touch with one of these, contact the Irish Women's Abortion Support Group in London (see page 195).

Methods of abortion

These vary according to how many weeks pregnant you are.

FIRST 3 TO 5 DAYS

For emergency or morning-after birth control methods, see pages 110 and 114.

FIRST 14 DAYS

No one can be certain they're pregnant until their period is about a week late. But menstrual extraction, sometimes called interception, can be used to take out all the contents of the womb within the first fourteen days after unprotected intercourse. In America it's used for 'lunch-time' abortions – it only takes a couple of hours of your time.

UP TO 12 WEEKS

The most common method used is called vacuum aspiration. A thin flexible plastic tube called a cannula is pushed up the vagina, through the cervix and into the womb. The other end is attached to a suction machine which draws the contents of the womb out. You may stay in overnight, or you may be able to leave after a few hours if the clinic or hospital has an out-patient service.

12 TO 16 WEEKS

At this stage you may be given a minor operation called a Dilation and Curettage (D and C). This is almost always done under a general anaesthetic. The cervix is stretched (or dilated) and the contents of the womb are scraped out (or curetted). You'll probably stay in overnight.

AFTER 16 WEEKS

Injections of salt solution or drugs can be used to make the womb contract so that it pushes out its contents. It creates a sort of mini-labour which can last several hours. You won't be given a general anaesthetic, but will be sedated so that you won't really be aware of what is happening. You stay in hospital for two or three days.

18 WEEKS ONWARDS

A hysterotomy (not a hysterectomy, which means removal of the womb) is an operation which involves cutting through the abdomen and the wall of the womb to remove the contents. It leaves a scar and should only be done at a late stage of pregnancy if other methods are not possible. You have to stay in the hospital or clinic for about a week and two to three weeks' convalescence is recommended afterwards.

After the abortion

Most women recover from their abortions very quickly. A general anaesthetic can leave you feeling quite tired for a day or two, but a little rest is all that's needed. Late abortions take longer to recover from. You may need a couple of days in bed. After a hysterotomy you should have a couple of weeks' rest to recover fully.

It's normal to bleed and feel cramp pains for several days afterwards. Use a sanitary towel, not a tampon, because it's very easy to get an infection if you push anything up your vagina. Don't have intercourse for six weeks. Avoid energetic exercise for a couple of weeks – or longer if your doctor tells you. If you're at school and have to take part in sports, or if your job is very strenuous, ask the doctor who arranged the abortion to write a note to get you excused – no reason need be given. Don't go swimming for six weeks.

Most doctors, clinics and hospitals arrange an appointment for a final check-up six weeks after an abortion. It's important to keep this appointment because it's possible that there will be a complication, although the majority of girls don't have any complications at all. Go to your doctor, clinic or hospital if you get a fever, very bad cramps or if the normal bleeding that happens after an abortion lasts for longer than ten days. If you suddenly start to bleed very heavily, get immediate medical attention. You can expect your first period from four to six weeks afterwards. If it doesn't come by this time, go to your doctor. If you do get an infection it has to be treated quickly but can be quite easily cured with antibiotics.

Many women feel relieved after their abortion. It's also quite normal to feel rather sad or depressed either immediately after the abortion or a few months later when the baby would have been born. This may also be like the depression many women feel after childbirth. It's partly a result of the changing level of hormones that takes place in the body of every woman after she's been pregnant – a natural feeling and it does go away. Or it may be because at any other time, under different circumstances, you would have liked a baby. Again, these feelings usually fade.

If you do feel upset – you may feel angry, lonely or guilty – don't bottle it up. It often helps to talk about it with a friend, especially one who's been through it all herself. You might find it helpful to go to a women's centre if there's one in your area (see page 201) or talk to the doctor or counsellor who arranged your abortion.

CHAPTER ELEVEN

Having a Baby

If you're having a baby you have to make several decisions – among them whether to live with the father of the baby, or marry him, or neither. Our society doesn't make it easy for a single girl to be pregnant or for anyone to bring up a child on their own. But there's no reason why anyone should go through it literally on her own. You may get a lot of support from your parents. But they may not know what to do either. There are many organizations (see page 196) which exist for no other reason than to help young unmarried girls with the problems they may have to face when they're pregnant. *Remember*: don't go it alone – you don't have to. These organizations are there to help you, so contact them.

Where to stay

A big problem facing pregnant girls whose parents are too shocked or angry to help is finding somewhere to stay. Being lonely will only make your pregnancy all the worse, especially if it's an unwanted pregnancy. Even if your parents are very upset, shocked or angry, unless you decide to live with the father of the baby it is probably best in the long run if you can stay at home – especially if you're under 18. Failing that, see if you can stay with a sympathetic friend or relative. Many of the organizations mentioned on page 196 will help you find somewhere to stay if you have to leave home.

If you feel you need somewhere to stay in the last couple of months of your pregnancy and immediately after the baby is born you may be able to go to a mother and baby home or live with a family. To find out about these possibilities, contact

144 · Make it Happy, Make it Safe

the National Council for One Parent Families (page 197), or the social services department of your local council (outside the cities, the social services are run by county authorities). Look them up in the phone directory or ask at the Town Hall.

Leaving home

If things do get really bad at home many girls decide to leave. Probably one of the unkindest things they can do is just to take off and leave their parents to worry themselves sick about where they are and what's happening to them. It's always worth ringing home to let your parents know that you're at least alive and well.

If you're under 18, your parents can legally ask the authorities to find you and bring you home. If you are found and if the social services department of the local council decides you are in need of 'care and protection', they can apply for a Care Order. This means that you will appear in court and the magistrates may appoint a social worker to decide whether you should live at home or in a residential or foster home. A Care Order passed when you are under 16 lasts until you are 18; if you're over 16 it lasts until you are 19. You can apply to the court at any time for the order to be ended. To find out how to do this contact the National Council for Civil Liberties (page 188), the Children's Legal Centre (page 187) or ask at your local Citizens Advice Bureau (look it up in the phone book).

When you are pregnant and under a Care Order, the social worker is involved in deciding what to do about your pregnancy. If you're under 16 you can't get an abortion without the consent of the social services department. But you have the right to decide whether to keep the baby or have it adopted or fostered. If you have any complaints about or problems with the social services department, contact the National Council for One Parent Families (page 197).

Medical care

It's very important for every pregnant girl or woman to look after her health and have regular medical attention particularly by the time she's fifteen weeks pregnant. (That's fifteen weeks after the day the last period started.)

You can register with any doctor who's prepared to take you on to her or his 'panel'. You can get a list of doctors in the area where you're staying from the local post office. If the doctors you contact all seem to be full up, ask for advice at the Citizens Advice Bureau. If your doctor doesn't offer a maternity service, she or he may send you to a doctor who does, or to a local clinic (called ante-natal clinics – ante-natal means before birth) which are often attached to hospitals.

If you're under 16 a doctor can't legally treat you without your parents' permission (except in emergencies). But much depends on what the doctor thinks: many believe that it is better to treat a young patient than to frighten them away and make them feel too scared ever to come for medical treatment.

You shouldn't be treated any differently whether you're married or single. At the clinic or hospital you'll probably be called 'Mrs' – the more enlightened ones will use just your first name. If you run into any problems about the way you're treated, contact the National Council for One Parent Families or the Patients Association.

Some hospitals have a medical social worker attached to them who can help patients sort out their practical problems, such as where to stay, money, and personal worries.

Finding out about pregnancy and childbirth

Doctors and clinics usually have a mass of leaflets about all aspects of pregnancy – diet, exercise, welfare rights, etc. – just ask for them. One Parent Families, the Family Planning Association and the National Childbirth Trust will answer any specific questions you have and they all produce many very helpful books and leaflets. Send for booklists. One of the best books to read is *Your Body, Your Baby, Your Life*, by Angela Phillips (Pandora Press, paperback).

Living together (cohabitation)

If you are over 16 but under 18 you can live together as long as you have the permission of your parents or legal guardians. If they won't give their permission, they can prevent you from living together by making you a Ward of Court (which means that you have to get the permission of the court to live together) or you may be put into the care of the local authority.

The legal and practical advantages and disadvantages of living together and of getting married are set out very clearly in *Women's Rights: A Practical Guide*, by Anna Coote and Tess Gill (Penguin, paperback).

Marriage

You can't get married until you're 16. If you live in England, Wales or Northern Ireland you need the written permission of your parents or legal guardians until you're 18 if you want to get married in a registry office. For a church ceremony you don't need any consent, provided you're both 16 or over and the banns are read on three consecutive Sundays without objection. In Scotland, you don't need any permission once you're 16. In the Republic of Ireland you need permission up to the age of 21.

Traditionally, couples over 16 but under 18 who can't get permission have eloped to Scotland. Gretna Green, the town nearest to the English border, became famous for so-called 'shotgun' marriages. But eloping to Scotland isn't such a very good idea. Scottish law insists that one or other of you lives for at least fifteen days in Scotland before you can marry. This usually gives parents and guardians enough time to make you a Ward of Court and a summons will be served on you telling you to appear in court. If you go ahead with the wedding, having received this summons, your marriage will still be legal but you may be prosecuted for contempt of court. This will mean that you'll have to attend a session in court for a legal ticking off. If you manage to get married without your parents' consent by lying about your age, your marriage will still be legal (providing you're over 16) but you could be prosecuted for making a false statement.

In most cases it's probably best to stay put and apply directly to the court for permission to marry. You'll need to go to the Clerk's office at your local Magistrates Court or County Court (look them up in the phone book) to get the necessary forms. Once you've filled these in and sent them back to the court you'll be told of the time, place and date of the hearing. Your case will be held in private although your parents will be allowed in. All you have to do is tell the magistrate why you want to marry. To find out if you can get legal aid to pay the costs, get a form from any solicitor, the Citizens Advice Bureau or the nearest Law Society Legal Aid Area Office (look them up in the phone book).

Adoption and fostering

Adoption means having your baby but then allowing it to be brought up by another family and giving up all your rights as a parent. Fostering means having your baby but then allowing it to be cared for either by another family or in a home, until you're able to look after it yourself.

Every mother has the right to decide for herself whether to keep her baby or have it adopted or fostered. The baby's father has no such rights. It's never an easy decision. You don't have to decide until after the baby is born, but it's a good idea to try to work it out in your own mind before. Many women feel differently after the birth. You have to be very careful not to make an unrealistic decision at a time when you might be feeling very strongly either way. Don't try to work it all out on your own – and don't be pressured into doing what you don't want to do. It's a big step in anyone's life and you'll need as much moral support and sympathy as you can get. The National Council for One Parent Families will give you all the advice, information and help you need on weighing up the argument for and against keeping your child, adoption or fostering. They won't put any pressure on you one way or the other. They'll also tell you about any similar organizations in your area.

Adoption and fostering can be arranged either through the social services department of your local council (look it up in phone book) or through one of the organizations listed on page 196. The British Agency for Adoption and Fostering can send you a list and advise you on agencies in your area.

Education

By law you have to be educated until you reach school-leaving age, which is 16. You may be able to stay on at your own school if you, your parents and the head teacher all agree. You may be able to transfer to another school nearby. In the past most schools used to expel any girl who became pregnant but many now have a more liberated and sympathetic approach. If you're under 16 and do leave school because you're pregnant, the local education authority has an obligation to make arrangements for a tutor to teach you at home or wherever you're staying. The minimum is ten hours a week but you may be able to get extra teaching if you're taking exams. Some authorities, however, don't have enough teachers and many girls find it difficult to get enough tuition to bring them up to exam-passing standards. In some areas there are special centres where pregnant schoolgirls can carry on learning if they're under 16. Ask your local education office whether there's one in your area.

Similar arrangements can be made if you're over 16 and want to stay on at school or college. Your head teacher or the welfare officer of the local education authority (look them up in the phone book or ask at the Town Hall) can help you and your parents with any education problems. If you run into any difficulties contact the National Council for One Parent Families (address, page 197) or the Advisory Centre for Education (address, page 189).

It may not be plain sailing but it is worth going on with your schooling. Getting pregnant shouldn't be a reason for giving up an education. Any girl who decides to keep her baby might well need the better money that often goes with a job that requires exam certificates, and it's never easy to pick up again once you've left off.

Work

A girl who has worked for the same employer for at least two years can't be sacked simply because she's pregnant. Any girl who has worked in the same job for less than two years but over six months and is sacked because she's pregnant may be able to take her case to the Tribunal for Unfair Dismissal. She will probably win her case unless her pregnancy has made it impossible for her to do her job (such as lifting very heavy loads, etc.) or if her job is too dangerous for a pregnant woman to do (such as working with X-rays or with certain chemicals). Some firms now give their workers paid leave for a month or two while they have their baby and just after, but they don't have to by law, so many don't. A few firms give their men workers paid leave while their wife or girlfriend has a baby.

Until the law makes it possible for women to insist on the right to maternity leave, and makes it impossible for firms to sack a worker just because she's pregnant, there's no doubt that many pregnant women will find themselves discriminated against. Obviously even if the law is not on their side, many firms will make life very unpleasant for someone they want to sack. This is certainly one area in which women still have to win some basic rights. In the meantime, anyone with work problems should try not to get too discouraged. In a time of high unemployment it's worth hanging on to your job until the last possible moment – but keep an eye open for any jobs that might be going.

Anyone with problems about being sacked or getting time off for medical treatment can get advice from One Parent Families or the Equal Opportunities Commission.

Money

To find out about grants, allowances, sickness, unemployment and supplementary benefits, etc., contact the local Department of Health and Social Security (look it up in the phone book). The Citizens Advice Bureau will also be able to give help on this matter. To claim these benefits and allowances you have to fill in various forms. Some of these forms are available from your local post office, others from the social security office. The post office should be able to tell you what to do; the Citizens Advice Bureau will help you fill them in. The Claimants Union (address, page 188) will also help you with information on what to claim for and how.

If you're at college you may be entitled to an extra allowance. To find out about this, contact the National Council for One Parent Families.

But remember, it's never enough. Having a baby costs a lot.

Rights of the father

A single mother is automatically her child's only legal guardian; the single father has no automatic rights over his child unless he gets them established in a court of law. It can be very difficult for a man to prove that he is the father of his child. If you want to take responsibility for your child and the mother refuses to let you, you will have to apply to the Magistrates Court. In court you have to prove that the mother accepted payments or gifts from you shortly after the baby was born and/or that she admitted that you were the father, perhaps in a letter or by telling people who you could then use as witnesses. A blood test to check out both your blood group and that of the baby can only prove that you are *not* the father of a child – it can't prove that you definitely are the father.

If the court decides that you are the father you will be responsible for supporting the child. If the mother of your child tries to prevent you from seeing your child you can apply to the Magistrates Court for 'right of access'. The court will probably rule that you should be allowed to see your child unless it decides that your character is so bad that it would be dangerous for the child if you did.

If you want to look after your child long term you will have to go to court and prove that the mother is incapable of looking after your child and that you are capable. In the past, courts have almost automatically assumed that a mother is better at looking after children than a father, however good he would be or however bad she might be at doing so. More and more courts are treating the mother and father as equals and deciding on the merits of each particular case – although most still decide in favour of the mother.

If you need any legal advice on the matter of paternity, contact a solicitor or the National Council for One Parent Families.

Maintenance

If the father refuses to accept responsibility and the mother wants him to support the child financially, she has to take 'affiliation proceedings' against him. This means going to a Magistrates Court and proving that he really is the father. You can apply for an affiliation order before the baby is born or up to three years after. You can't apply if you are married to another man and are living with him. You don't *have* to claim maintenance from the father if you don't want to. If you are claiming social security, you may be under some pressure to accept maintenance because this means you get less money from the social security. You don't have to tell them who the father is or where he is.

CHAPTER TWELVE

Make It Healthy

When we're young our parents are always telling us to clean our teeth, scrub our nails, wash behind our ears, not to go out with wet hair, etc., etc. – probably until we're sick of it. But they hardly ever tell us much about how we should look after our genitals. As a result, some of us don't take enough care about the health of our genitals and others worry too much. Even reading about the different illnesses that are around can make us feel convinced that we've caught some dreadful disease. (It's even worse when you're writing about them!) But, apart from herpes which needn't be very serious, and AIDS which *is* very serious, diseases of the sex organs are fairly easy to cure and most are easy to prevent.

It's as important to tell the difference between healthy and unhealthy sex organs as it is for any other part of our body. If we don't keep them clean and look after them, they can get infected and will need medical treatment.

A healthy vagina naturally produces a small amount of clear or slightly milky discharge. These fluids are produced in order to keep the sensitive skin around the vagina soft and moist. This discharge may be slightly heavier – and sometimes a bit yellowish – just before a period. If a girl or woman doesn't wash her genitals every day they will get musty and sweaty like any other part of her body.

Boys also produce a natural secretion which, if he's uncircumcised (i.e. still has a foreskin), collects under his foreskin. This is called smegma and is usually a yellowish-whitish colour. A circumcised penis may also produce traces of smegma. If this isn't washed away every day it can start to smell a bit high.

All you need to keep your genitals clean is soap and water.

Jokes about cunts that smell like fish and cocks that smell like overripe cheese don't help to make us feel very confident about our normal, healthy, natural personal smells. Don't be taken in by adverts for vaginal deodorants or heavily scented soaps and powders. In order to sell their products, the makers would have us believe that our genitals are somehow 'dirty' and that their natural smell is 'offensive'. It's simply not true. Many lovers find that their partner's smells are something of a turn-on. Deodorants make us all smell the same and can cause irritations.

There are some basic rules for keeping our genitals clean and healthy:

—Wash your genitals every day.
—After going to the loo, wipe your bottom from the front to the back.
—Wash yourself thoroughly after having sex.
—If you use the cap for contraception, wash it really well after use and dust it with talcum powder.
—Don't put anything into the vagina or anus that you think might have germs on it.

There are several illnesses that you can get by having sex with someone who has an infection. These are called sexually transmitted diseases. There are also some illnesses that affect the sex organs that don't come about as a result of having sex. But you can pass these on to your partner. This means two things: if your partner does have an infection you can't assume that she or he has necessarily been sleeping with someone else. It also means that, however you got your infection, you must go to a doctor to get it cured.

One reason why there is such a lot of sexually transmitted disease around is that those suffering from one are often made to feel guilty so they daren't go to a doctor to get better. This is a bit strange if you think about it. No one blames a person for getting flu or any other illness. But when it comes to infections that affect the sex organs, many people react by thinking 'Serves you right for having sex', or 'She/he must be putting it around a lot.' These reactions probably have a lot to do with people's attitudes about sex. If you don't think of sex as a perfectly normal part of living (which it certainly is) or if you think that sex with more than one person during the whole of your life is wrong (which it certainly needn't be), then you can see why some people will think of a sexually transmitted disease as some sort of divine punishment for being 'dirty', 'naughty' or 'sinful'. But no illness is a punishment. The Christian Church does not believe that God punishes people by making them ill. (If they believed this, then Christians would have to see all other diseases, such as diabetes or multiple sclerosis, as a punishment.) And a sexually transmitted disease is not caught by being 'naughty', or by having sex with a great number of different people. You get it merely by having sex with just one person who happens to be infected with the disease.

Because in the early days of AIDS the majority of sufferers from this disease in the USA and in Europe were gay, the popular press were able to exploit a general ignorance and fear of the disease to stir up a disgusting and repulsive anti-gay panic and hysteria. Gays everywhere, whether or not they had AIDS, were shunned and treated barbarically. One American politician was overheard to say that his cure for AIDS was to 'shoot all queers'. Extreme prejudice like this is just as harmful as the disease – it may prove to be even more difficult to cure than AIDS itself. We now know that AIDS is not a 'gay plague' as it was once described. For a start, it isn't only an illness that gays suffer from – anyone can get it. Secondly, it isn't a plague. You can't get AIDS from simply being near someone with the infection, as you could catch the plague. But AIDS has shown us that many people who think that a disease which can be sexually transmitted is some sort of punishment are less worried about curing illnesses, and more interested in trying to stamp out all sex that isn't between married couples. 'Down with illness' should be the slogan – not 'Down with sex.'

Prevention of disease

Many people who suffer from sexually transmitted diseases don't show any signs at all. You can't protect yourself merely by taking a look at your partner's genitals. But there are certain things you can do to try to avoid at least some of the illnesses.

—Keep your genitals clean. Washing before and after sex is a good idea.
—Limit your number of partners. You're obviously more likely to pick up a disease the more people you sleep with. The same is true if your partner has a number of different partners.
—Don't have sex with anyone who has any sores or rashes around their genitals.
—Avoid oral sex with someone who has cold sores on their mouths – you can give and get genital herpes this way. And the virus that can lead to AIDS may be transmitted this way too.
—No french kissing if either of you have sores in your mouth or bleeding gums. (Your gums can bleed if you floss your teeth too vigorously.) It is possible that the virus that can cause AIDS can be passed on by french kissing if there are any sores or scratches in either partner's mouth.
—If you decide to have intercourse rather than enjoying sex in other ways, use a condom plus spermicide (check page 114 on how to use one properly). Condoms are definitely a part of safer sex, but they can split.
—Use a spermicide with Nonoxynol in it. This helps protect against AIDS as well as pregnancy.
—Don't go in for any sort of sex play that breaks the skin – such as biting or scratching.
—Don't have anal sex. Condoms are much more likely to split during anal sex than during vaginal sex. In some parts of the world anal sex is the main way in which the virus causing AIDS is transmitted.

—Some infections such as cystitis and urethritis can be prevented if you pee immediately after having sex.
—If the vagina is a bit dry or feels sore buy some lubricating jelly from the chemist, such as KY Jelly. You don't need a prescription. Many couples find this useful when they use condoms.
—Many genital infections can be prevented or controlled if you wear cotton rather than nylon pants, baggy trousers rather than tight ones, and stockings rather than tights.
—Scented soap and bath oils can cause irritations and infection. Stick to simple plain soap.

General symptoms

Here are some to look out for:

—an unusual discharge from the vagina or tip of the penis
—sores, blisters, rashes or irritation in or around the vagina, anus or penis
—pain or a hot burning feeling when you pee
—wanting to pee very often
—blood in your pee
—pain while you're having sex
—any unusual lump or bump – that may not even be painful.

If you suffer from any of these symptoms then the chances are that you have some sort of infection. You should not have sex until you have been to see a doctor. But not all people suffer from any of these signs, even though they have an infection. If a partner suffers from any of these symptoms you should definitely go to a doctor yourself as well. Remember, it doesn't have to mean that your partner has been sleeping with anyone else. Either of you might have picked up an infection in an earlier relationship but not shown any symptoms.

Where to get treatment

You can go to your family doctor, but some sexually transmitted diseases need specialist medical knowledge which
your own doctor may not have. There are special clinics in
most cities and towns which deal with all sexually transmitted diseases. These aren't the grim places they once were.
You can go to any special clinic for free advice and treatment.
You don't need a letter from your family doctor. You may
need to make an appointment, so ring up first. All treatment
is absolutely confidential. They are called by a variety of
different names: Special Clinic, Department of Genito-
urinary Medicine, Department of Venereology, STD Clinic,
Department of Genital Medicine.

To find your nearest clinic, look it up in the phone book
under any of these names. Or it might be listed under
Venereal Disease. Or you can phone your local hospital; the
hospital operator should be able to tell you where to go. You
can also ask a Citizens Advice Bureau or family planning
clinic. (It would make life a lot easier if they were all called by
the same name.)

Go along to the clinic with your partner – she or he will
need an appointment too, and it's always better to share a
problem. Or go with a friend. It's a good idea to give your real
name and address to avoid confusion. And these clinics are
totally discreet, absolutely confidential – and they've treated
thousands of young people who have felt a bit scared. They're
really not such awful places to go to.

AT THE CLINIC

A woman or girl shouldn't make an appointment for when
she's having her period because some of the tests won't work
too well at this time of the month. You'll be asked the
following questions:

—your name, address and date of birth

—brief details about your medical history – what illnesses you've had and so on
—whether you're allergic to any particular medicines
—whether you are – or might be – pregnant
—why you've come to the clinic – what symptoms you have or what your worries are
—some specific details about the sort of sexual contact you've had (if any), whether you've had oral, vaginal or anal sex.

After this you'll have to give a urine sample and a blood test and you'll be given an examination. For this you'll have to undress from the waist down. You may find this embarrassing, especially if you haven't done it before. But no one in these clinics is going to judge you. They're there to help you get better. They're against illness, not against sex.

Smear samples will then be taken. For a girl, this involves lying on her back with her legs apart; the doctor or nurse will insert an instrument called a speculum into her vagina which holds the walls of the vagina apart to allow a little wooden or plastic spatula to scrape some cells from her cervix. Swabs may also be taken from her anus, pee-hole and throat.

For a boy, a swab is taken by gently placing a tiny loop or cotton wool swab a little way into the hole in the tip of his penis. This may sound horrific but most say they hardly feel a thing. Smears may also be taken from his anus and throat. Some samples will be looked at under the microscope while you wait, others will go to a laboratory and you won't get the results for several days or maybe longer.

You won't be given a test for the virus that causes AIDS unless you ask for one (see page 165). And a girl won't be tested for possible cancer of her cervix. Nor will you be tested automatically for herpes or chlamydia. If you are worried about any of these, mention it to the doctor.

Because it can be something of a nerve-wracking experience, you might find that you forget to ask about the things that are really worrying you. Some people find it a good idea to write out their questions on a bit of paper beforehand.

REMEMBER

—The first visit may take up to an hour or even longer if there is a long queue.

—You may have to go back for more visits before correct treatment is given.

—If you need to take time off from school, college or work you can ask for a doctor's certificate of attendance. This won't say why you're there.

—Everything that happens at these clinics is confidential. Your family doctor won't be told, nor will your parents, even if you're under 16.

—You don't have to give your age.

—Don't have sex with anyone until you've been told that you're completely cured.

—Once you have been cured you can catch the infection again if you have sex with someone who is infected. So if you have a regular partner, make sure he or she also goes to the clinic to get cured before you have sex with them.

Contact tracing

If everyone with a sexually transmitted disease went for treatment and told their partners that they could be infected, and they also went for treatment, these diseases would soon disappear. But too many people are made to feel guilty or ashamed to admit it – sometimes even to themselves. To try to prevent the spread of the more serious diseases such as AIDS, gonorrhoea and syphilis, many health authorities like to trace all those who have had sex with an infected person. This is why some clinics ask for the names of those you've recently had sex with. They then, very discreetly (or else no one would ever give them any names), get in touch with everyone who may have caught the disease. Their hope is that they will get in touch with contacts before they have sex with anyone else and so spread the disease even further.

You don't have to give the clinic any names if you don't want to. But if you decide not to, you really must tell everyone you think you might have caught the disease from or who you might have given the disease to. If you don't, and they never discover that they have the disease (not all diseases have any symptoms, so some people don't ever know that they're infected), they may not only give it to someone else but they, and many more besides, could become seriously ill and possibly end up unable to have babies – or dead.

Illnesses and sexually transmitted diseases

AIDS

AIDS stands for Acquired Immune Deficiency Syndrome. Acquired means that it's not something you are born with but an illness you catch. Immune refers to the body's immune system in the bloodstream which, when working properly, protects us from getting ill. Immune deficiency means that sufferers from AIDS are unable to protect themselves from any illness. A syndrome is a group of illnesses which help to identify a particular disease.

AIDS, then, is a disorder of the blood which causes the body's immune system to cease functioning properly. This disorder seems to be caused by a virus called HIV, which stands for Human Immunodeficiency Virus.

There is a difference between having HIV, the virus that can lead to AIDS, and having AIDS itself. HIV can stay in a person's bloodstream for years without them showing any signs or symptoms. The majority of people infected by the virus will remain well for a number of years, but they are able to transmit the disease to others. Once someone is infected with HIV, the virus will stay in their body for the rest of their life. Some people with HIV may develop illnesses such as swollen lymph glands, especially in the armpits or in the back of the neck, certain skin infections, and other symptoms such as thrush in their mouths, diarrhoea and general ill-health. People with these symptoms are said to have ARC which

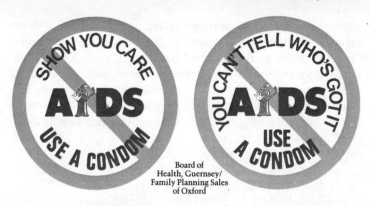

Board of
Health, Guernsey/
Family Planning Sales
of Oxford

stands for AIDS-Related Complex. They are more likely to go
on to get AIDS than those who have HIV and are well.

AIDS affects only a small proportion of people infected
with HIV. An AIDS sufferer develops certain infections and
cancers which will probably eventually kill them. Because
the body's immune system has been knocked out by HIV the
body cannot throw off these illnesses. Such illnesses are
called 'opportunistic' infections, which means that in a
healthy body they are harmless, but in the body of someone
with HIV they take the opportunity provided by the absence
of an immune system that normally works to destroy disease.
The most common opportunistic infections in AIDS sufferers are a type of pneumonia, infections of the gut, various
neurological disorders, and tumours, especially a cancer
called Kaposi's sarcoma.

SYMPTOMS

It's difficult to give a complete list of symptoms because no
two people with either the virus that can lead to AIDS or with
AIDS itself are alike. People with HIV may not have any
symptoms at all – or not for several months or years after they
are infected. Someone with ARC may have very bad symptoms or quite mild ones which come and go. People suffering
from AIDS itself will all be seriously ill and will probably
eventually die from one or other of the opportunistic infections and cancers.

Some symptoms to watch out for are: a sudden loss of weight; swollen glands; sweating and flu-like symptoms for longer than a couple of weeks; purplish or dark brown blotches anywhere on your body; a persistent cough that won't go away.

But all or any of these symptoms don't necessarily mean that you've got HIV or AIDS. It may just mean that you've got glandular fever and/or flu and/or a bad cough. But if you are worried, either go to your doctor or a clinic and ask for advice.

HOW THE VIRUS THAT CAN LEAD TO AIDS
IS TRANSMITTED

You can't get AIDS that easily. It's not like flu or the common cold which you can get merely by being in the same room as someone with the illness. The AIDS virus is actually rather delicate and can't live outside the body. Outside the body it is easily killed by bleach or strong household disinfectants, or by extreme heat or cold.

The HIV virus that can lead to AIDS damages the body's immune system by attacking a particular group of cells in the bloodstream. To do this the virus has to get into the blood either directly from the blood of an infected person or from various body fluids which can contain the virus, such as urine, menstrual blood, semen, faeces (shit), vaginal secretions, breast milk and possibly saliva.

Intercourse, both vaginal and anal, is the most common way HIV is transmitted from one person to another. The virus in an infected person is found in his semen and her vaginal secretions and menstrual blood. During intercourse the virus can pass into the bloodstream of the partner being penetrated, either through small cuts and tears in the vagina or anus which happen quite normally during intercourse, or by being absorbed through the walls of the passage inside the anus (called the rectum) or vagina. It is also possible for the virus to pass from the person being penetrated from the fluids inside their vagina or rectum into the penis of the person who is penetrating.

This tells us quite a number of things. Firstly, that anyone can get the HIV virus that can lead to AIDS. It isn't just homosexuals who can get AIDS. It also tells us that intercourse without a condom and a spermicide containing Nonoxynol, which destroys the virus, is definitely unsafe. But more than this, it tells us that the virus cannot be passed from one person to another by simply touching, shaking hands, using someone else's musical instrument, drinking out of the same glass, using the same telephone or laundrette, from swimming pools, or by sharing toilet or canteen facilities etc. Mosquitoes can't pass on the virus either.

Traces of the virus have also been found in other body fluids, such as tears, and mucus in the nose. But teardrops or mucus from the nose, say from a big spluttery sneeze, would have to fall directly on to an open cut and in very large quantities for there to be any likelihood of getting the virus.

Drug addicts who inject drugs directly into their veins (called intravenous or IV drug-users) are highly likely to get the virus unless they make absolutely certain that every needle they use is absolutely clean and hasn't been used by anyone else. When an IV drug-user injects herself or himself, a bit of their blood goes back up into the needle. This blood then goes straight into the bloodstream of the next person to use the needle. Anyone who uses dirty works when injecting drugs is at very high risk of passing on and getting the virus. So are their sexual partners unless they practise safer sex.

Pregnant women who are infected with the virus are more likely to develop AIDS, which is why many doctors recommend an abortion as this may save their lives. There is a second reason: their babies are likely to be born with the virus and, because the immune system in a new-born baby is not very strong, they will probably develop AIDS and die. Mothers with the virus may be advised not to breastfeed their babies as it is possible that the virus can pass from the mother to the baby through her breast milk.

Oral sex and french kissing may also transmit the virus. Although this is probably fairly unlikely, it is possible that the virus could be passed on either by infected semen or by

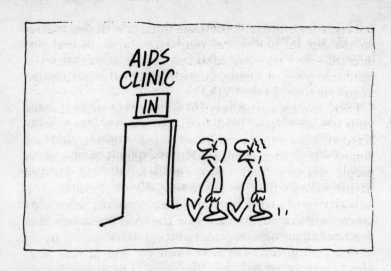

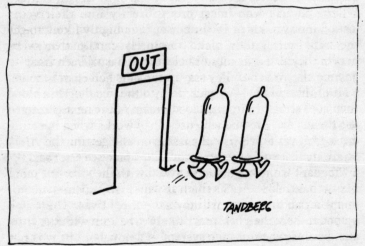

Gay or straight – safer sex means that everyone should be using condoms.

saliva getting into the bloodstream through scratches or sores on the mouth, lips, gums, tongue or throat. In oral sex, infected saliva could be absorbed by the membranes just inside the penis or vagina, through any small scratches that might be caused by the teeth.

There are some other ways in which it is known that the virus has been transmitted. In the past, before governments acted to help stamp out the disease, blood from infected blood donors was given to those needing blood transfusions. Many people suffering from a rare disease of the blood called haemophilia got the virus in this way. Blood in blood banks is now all treated so that you can't get the virus in this way any longer. All blood donors are now tested to make sure they don't have the virus.

THE HIV ANTIBODY TEST

When the HIV virus first gets into the bloodstream, the person may not know she or he has the infection for months or maybe years. But the blood tries to destroy the infection by making some antibodies. These don't actually manage to destroy the virus but they stay in the blood and can be found by examining a blood sample. They don't show up in a blood test until about three months after the infection has entered the body.

This means that while there is no way of testing for AIDS itself or for the HIV virus, you can be tested for the HIV antibodies. If these are found you can tell whether or not a person has the HIV virus that can cause AIDS. It doesn't tell you whether the person will go on to get AIDS. But it does tell you that she or he *must* practise safer sex to make sure their partner doesn't get the virus. And because you can never be absolutely sure that your partner doesn't have the virus, you should practise safer sex anyway.

There are some drawbacks about having the test done. Although the clinic will keep the result absolutely confidential, some people who are antibody positive are being refused life insurance, mortgages, and even hospital treatment (even though nobody who has looked after a patient either with the virus or with AIDS has ever got the disease by looking after them – except in a few cases where a nurse or doctor has accidentally jabbed themselves with a needle that had been used by the patient). Others have found that, because people are both ignorant and scared about AIDS, if they are antibody positive their friends, family, and fellow workers refuse to come anywhere near them. If you decide you want the test, you will talk over all the arguments for and against with a doctor or health worker at the clinic first. If you want to have a baby, you may think it's a good idea for both you and your partner to be tested to be on the safe side.

PREVENTION

The very fact of having lots of different sex partners doesn't give you the virus. But the law of averages means that the more partners you have, the more likely you are to come across someone who is infected. However, you can sleep with just one person who might have it. So, while cutting down on the number of partners is a good idea, you're not automatically safe just because you have only one partner.

Safer sex, then, means the following:

—Don't have any sex that allows his or her blood (including menstrual blood), semen, urine, vaginal secretions, or faeces (shit) to enter your vagina, anus or mouth or touch your penis. Without any doubt, penetrative sex, that is sex in which his penis enters your vagina, anus or mouth, is the most dangerous thing to do. If you really must have sex in this way, *always* use a condom and a spermicide foam, jelly or cream with Nonoxynol in it. This kills the virus on contact. Don't be tempted to use just a condom or just a spermicide. AIDS is too dangerous to take any risks.

—Don't go in for french kissing if either of you have any sores or cuts in or around the mouth.

—Think about all the other ways of enjoying sex that don't involve any risks. Masturbating each other (check there are no cuts or sores on either of your bodies – if there are, cover them with waterproof plasters) can be a lovely, warm way in which to share sexual pleasure.

—Rubbing or massaging each other's bodies with a deliciously scented oil (or baby oil will do) is another way of giving and getting pleasure.

—You'll need to know something about the sexual history of your partner. Being open and honest is a definite must if we are to stamp out this disease. If you can't talk freely with your partner, don't take any chances at all.

—Don't share razors or toothbrushes.

—Unless you are absolutely certain that all their equipment is sterilized or new each time it's used, don't have your ears pierced, and don't get tattooed. If you go to an acupuncturist or have any hair removed by electrolysis, make sure they use sterilized equipment. If they're any good at their job, they won't mind you discussing this.

—It's extremely unlikely that you could get the virus at the dentist's. But to protect themselves as well as their patients, dentists should wear surgical gloves.

—Don't share your works with anyone if you are an IV drug-user.

CURE

There is no cure for either the HIV virus or for AIDS itself. The HIV virus may not develop into AIDS – but the person with the virus can pass it on to someone else who might go on to get AIDS. Anyone with AIDS itself will probably eventually die from one of the infections that form the syndrome. It's the most serious sexually transmitted disease that we currently face.

CANDIDA ALBICANS
(also called thrush, monilias yeast infection, candidosis or candidiasis)

Yeast or fungus grows normally in the vagina, but is usually kept under control by the acid content of the natural vaginal secretions. If your system is thrown off balance, the yeast starts to grow uncontrollably. This infection is sometimes not sexually transmitted at all – although it can be. The contraceptive pill can cause it for some girls and women. So can certain antibiotics that you may be taking for some other infection. Borrowed towels, swimwear and pants can spread it from one person to another. A baby can pick up thrush in its mouth if its mother has thrush when it's being born.

SYMPTOMS

For girls, thrush produces a thick white vaginal discharge which looks like cottage cheese and smells like baking bread. It makes you feel very itchy inside your vagina and painful when you pee. In boys, thrush may not be so noticeable, but can cause irritation and soreness under the foreskin.

TREATMENT

The doctor will prescribe tablets that you push into your vagina (called pessaries) and/or a special cream. Cotton underwear, sanitary towels and not tampons, and utmost cleanliness will help it go away more quickly. Some girls and women find that live natural plain yoghurt pushed up into the vagina helps lessen the itchiness.

PREVENTION

Sexual intercourse using either a condom or cap should prevent thrush in many cases. If a girl seems to get it quite often, she should always ask her doctor for an antibiotic that won't cause thrush. Use a sanitary towel rather than a tampon until all symptoms have gone away.

CANCER

If it is discovered early enough, cancer can be cured in the majority of cases. Sadly, not everyone realizes this and, perhaps because the very thought of cancer is so frightening, many people don't go for the necessary treatment at the stage when they could be cured. Regular checking for breast cancer and cancer of the testicles, and screening for cancer of the cervix, ought to be an essential part of how we look after our health.

Cancer occurs when some cells in a part of our body start to multiply uncontrollably. If this happens near the outside of our body, we can feel a lump. Eventually the cancerous cells get into the bloodstream and travel to other organs inside the body. If it is to be cured, cancer must be discovered before this spread is allowed to happen.

BREAST CANCER

Both females and males can get breast cancer, although it's more frequently found in women. It's a good idea for girls to get used to making regular examinations of their breasts. The best time to do this is just after a period.

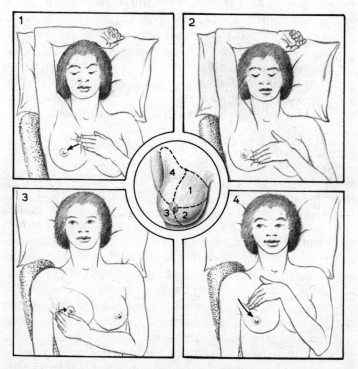

Breast self-examination: get into the habit of checking your breasts regularly for any early signs of cancer.

What you do is this. First of all, standing up, look in a mirror as you check what they look like. See if there are any changes in size (most girls and women have breasts that are a bit different from each other in size and shape). Gently squeeze each nipple just in case there is any bleeding or discharge. Then, lying down with one arm up behind your head, examine the right breast with your left hand. Massage the whole breast in a circular fashion, moving from the outside towards the nipple with the flat of the tips of your middle three fingers. Then do your other breast with your other hand. Breasts are naturally lumpy so don't think that every lump or ridge means that you have cancer. Regular self-examination will soon make you familiar with the normal masses and, should an abnormal lump appear, you'll know immediately and can get it checked out by your doctor.

If you discover any abnormal lump, any bleeding or discharge, don't wait, hoping that it will go away. You may not have cancer at all, but only a harmless cyst that may not even need any treatment. But check it out – your doctor will either be able to set your mind at rest or be able to treat you in the early stages while the cancer is relatively harmless.

CANCER OF THE CERVIX (CERVICAL CANCER)

The cervix is right deep inside your vagina. It's also called the neck of the womb or uterus. There are probably several causes of cancer of the cervix. Doctors have noticed that it's more likely to occur in girls and women who have the genital wart virus which is sexually transmitted. The same is true in girls and women who have other sexually transmitted diseases such as genital herpes and chlamydia. Those who started having sex at a young age during their teens, especially if they didn't use either the condom or cap, also seem to be at greater risk. And it seems to be related to the younger the girl is when she has a baby – it's more common among women who have had children in their teens. Smoking seems to be connected too. Nicotine passes from the bloodstream to the mucus that covers the cervix and destroys the immune system that protects against the disease.

If all or any of these things are true for you, you should go to your doctor and ask for a smear test. It doesn't mean that you'll necessarily get cervical cancer, but it does mean that you should have regular tests. It takes the cancer cells in your cervix from three to five years to develop. So a test every three years is an absolute must if you think you might be at some risk of getting this cancer. (Some doctors think that a test every five years is OK. More and more women are realizing that if they're at high risk this is too long to wait.)

The smear tests (also called Pap tests, or cyto tests) are fairly painless. Most girls and women say they feel more embarrassment than pain. You'll have to undress from the waist down and lie on a couch on your back with your legs apart. The doctor will gently insert something called a speculum into your vagina. This is made of plastic or metal and the doctor usually smears it with a slippery lubricating jelly to make it slide in more easily. A few cells will be gently scraped from the cervix with a small spatula or swab of cotton-wool on a little stick. Sometimes the doctor has to put her or his gloved finger into your anus in order to feel up further into your body than your vagina goes, in order to check from the inside how the womb feels.

The smear will then be sent to a laboratory. You'll be told when you can contact the doctor or clinic to find out the result of the test. They may write to let you know. But if you don't hear from them, call anyway just in case their letter has gone missing. Don't assume just because you haven't heard that there's nothing wrong.

If you are told that the test is positive, this means they have found some abnormal cells. This does not necessarily mean that you have cancer. Mild cell abnormality (called dysplasia) often goes back to normal without any treatment. All you'll have to do is go back for another smear test sooner than usual. If the cell change is a bit more serious you may be treated in the outpatients department of your local hospital with a local anaesthetic. Or you may be given a minor operation under a general anaesthetic. This usually means a stay of a few days in hospital. The surgeon will cut out a small area from the cervix about the size of a thumb nail. This will not affect a girl's sex life, or prevent her from having babies.

CANCER OF THE PENIS OR TESTICLES

This is fairly rare. Like all cancer, it must be treated in its early stages if it is to be cured. Any inflammation, difficulty in peeing, discharge, swelling, lump or spot or pain in the penis or balls should be reported to your doctor as soon as you've noticed it. It may be nothing more than a rupture or a harmless cyst. But only your doctor will be able to tell you.

CHLAMYDIA

(pronounced klam-id-eeah)

This is probably the most common sexually transmitted disease in the world. If left untreated in males it can cause NSU (see page 185) and in females it can lead to a much more serious illness called pelvic inflammatory disease (see page 182) which may result in infertility. So it's very important to get this disease treated quickly.

SYMPTOMS

Females rarely get any symptoms but if they do it may be as some discharge from the vagina. Males may get a discharge from the penis. Both may feel some pain when peeing and some irritation or soreness in the vagina or penis.

TREATMENT

If your partner has chlamydia, then the chances are that you have it too. But because there are often no symptoms at all it's difficult to tell. It often accompanies another sexually transmitted disease such as gonorrhoea. If you think it's possible that you have it (girls and women using the coil are especially vulnerable), go to the special clinic and ask to be tested. Not many doctors are clued up about chlamydia so you may have to insist on being tested. When discovered early enough, chlamydia is very easy to cure with antibiotics that you take in pill form.

PREVENTION

Sexual intercourse with a condom or cap will prevent it from being transmitted sexually.

CYSTITIS

This is a very common illness – probably as many as half of all girls and women suffer from it at some time in their lives. Cystitis is an infection of the bladder and its outlet tube, the urethra. It can be caused in a variety of different ways. Germs from the anus can get into the urethra in a girl or woman quite easily and this can cause cystitis. An allergy to certain perfumed soaps, bath salts and oils, or to vaginal deodorants, can also cause it. Cystitis after sexual intercourse – especially after the first time or two (cystitis is sometimes known as the 'honeymoon disease') – is fairly common. This is caused by bruising of the urethra by the penis during intercourse, because the urethra is so close to the inside of the vagina. Stress and illness can also bring on an attack in some women. More women get cystitis than men, but both can suffer from it and it can be sexually transmitted.

SYMPTOMS

Sufferers feel the need to pee very often, almost all the time, even though very little comes out. And when you do pee it is incredibly painful – a burning feeling. There may be blood or pus in your urine. You may also feel a pain and in the lower back.

TREATMENT

Sometimes the infection can spread to the kidneys and this makes it a more serious illness. Because of the risk to the kidneys, everyone who gets the symptoms should go to their doctor for advice. This is especially important for girls under 15 whose kidneys are still growing.

Your doctor will check the type of germs causing the infection from a sample of your pee which you'll be asked for at the surgery. Antibiotics or drugs called sulphonamides may be prescribed to kill the germs. You may need an X-ray to see if there is any kidney damage. While tests are being done the following will help:

—Keep up a good flushing-through effect by drinking at least five pints of water every day. Don't drink tea, coffee or alcohol.
—Pee frequently – at least six times a day.
—One bath a day is not enough. Keep a special flannel to wash round the entrance to the urethra each morning and evening and after you've been to the toilet. Don't use strong soaps, deodorants, antiseptics, creams or powder.
—If your symptoms are related to sexual intercourse and you get an attack regularly sometime during the forty-eight hours after intercourse, you may prevent attacks by the following: both partners wash their sex organs before intercourse with cool water: dry gently: use a lubricant such as K Y Jelly to prevent soreness and bruising: the girl should go to the toilet preferably fifteen minutes before intercourse and definitely within fifteen minutes after intercourse.
—If an attack starts, drink half a pint of water every twenty minutes. Each hour for three hours take a level teaspoon of bicarbonate of soda in water which will help lessen the burning feeling. Keep warm, and wash your vaginal area from front to back after every visit to the toilet. After these three hours the attack should have lessened sufficiently for you to go to your doctor.
—Avoid nylon underwear, tights and tight trousers.
—Hot water bottles on your tummy and against the lower part of your back may help to ease any pain.

PREVENTION

Try to learn what causes your attacks and follow the advice given above. A really good book called *Understanding Cystitis: A complete self-help guide* by Angela Kilmartin (Century-Arrow) will tell you all you need to know about helping to prevent cystitis.

GARDNERELLA
(anaerobic vaginosis)

This infection of the vagina isn't always transmitted sexually. Women and girls may have the germ for years without it becoming active. It's sometimes called by the general term non-specific vaginitis. (Any illness which ends in '-itis' means an inflammation.) Males can also get gardnerella, in which case it's usually called non-specific urethritis (NSU).

SYMPTOMS

A heavy, greyish, often fishy-smelling discharge from the vagina. There may be no symptoms at all – boys and men seldom get any symptoms, or they may feel some soreness when peeing.

TREATMENT

Your doctor or special clinic will prescribe a course of antibiotics in pill form.

PREVENTION

Sexual intercourse with a condom or cap will prevent it from being transmitted sexually.

GONORRHOEA

Gonorrhoea is one of three sexually transmitted diseases that are officially defined as venereal diseases. The others are syphilis and soft sore or chancre (this last venereal disease has disappeared in recent years). The term 'venereal' comes from the word Venus, the ancient goddess of love, which may sound like a bad joke to anyone suffering from a venereal disease. You can't catch a venereal disease (often shortened to VD) from swimming pools, toilet seats, towels or any way other than by direct sexual contact. This means either through anal or vaginal intercourse or by oral sex.

Gonorrhoea is the most common of venereal diseases. It's sometimes called 'the clap' or 'a dose'.

SYMPTOMS

The symptoms are different for females and males. In girls and women there are often no symptoms at all. In males the symptoms are usually obvious. If there are any symptoms

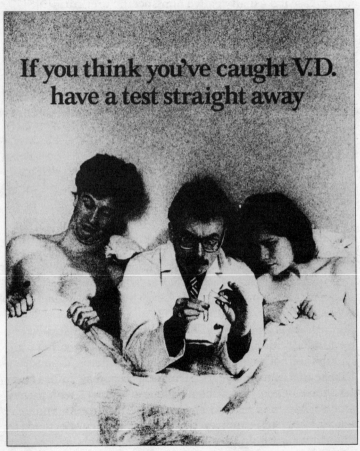

If you think you've caught V.D. have a test straight away

Sexually transmitted diseases (sometimes shortened to VD, which stands for venereal disease) can all be tested for at your local clinic.

these will show up from two to ten days after the infection has been caught. Women may get an unusual discharge, often yellowish, from the vagina. They may feel a burning feeling when peeing. They may get a slight fever, feel chill, and get some pains in the stomach and joints. They may be an infection in the anus which causes a discharge and irritation.

Men will probably feel pain when peeing, have a yellow discharge from the penis, and an irritation and discharge from the anus.

TREATMENT

If it's not treated, whether or not there are any symptoms, the gonorrhoea germs will spread to the rest of the internal sex organs and cause inflammation. Eventually, this could mean that it will be impossible ever to have a baby.

Treatment is simple: some tablets or one or more injections of an antibiotic in your bottom or thigh is all that's needed. You must go back to the clinic to check that it's been completely cured. Some strains of the gonorrhoea infection are proving harder to cure than others, but all this means is that the doctor has to give you a different antibiotic.

PREVENTION

Using a condom during intercourse prevents the spread of gonorrhoea. Doctors have noticed that gay men do not suffer from venereal diseases as much as they used to: this is because they are practising safer sex which helps prevent the spread of all diseases, not just AIDS.

HEPATITIS

The viruses causing hepatitis A and hepatitis B can be transmitted sexually. The virus is found in the sufferer's faeces (shit) and so is likely to be transmitted by anal intercourse and oral sex that involves the mouth coming into contact with the anus.

SYMPTOMS

Hepatitis attacks the liver and causes nausea, vomiting, jaundice and permanent liver damage. Hepatitis B is the most dangerous form because those who have recovered from it can continue to carry the virus in their body and can transmit it to their partner.

TREATMENT

A doctor can give injections of hepatitis B vaccine to protect the partner of someone who is carrying the virus. Until this has happened oral and anal sex should be avoided. The illness itself can't be cured.

PREVENTION

Safer sex – use a condom and avoid oral and anal sex – will protect you from hepatitis. Drug addicts who inject themselves should never share their works as this is another way in which hepatitis can be passed from one person to another.

HERPES

There are two common types of herpes. Herpes Type 1 is a virus that attacks the upper part of the body, usually forming cold sores around the mouth and nose. Herpes Type 2 usually forms sores around the genitals and anus. It is thought that the herpes virus usually gets to the genital area by oral sex, although it's perfectly possible for it to be spread if a person first touches the cold sore on their mouth and then touches their genitals. It can also be transmitted by having intercourse with someone who has a herpes sore on their genitals.

SYMPTOMS

The first attack of genital herpes is usually the worst. A really painful sore appears on the vagina, vulva, penis or anal area, often accompanied by a fever and general run down, flu-like symptoms. The sore will develop into swollen red blisters which burst, leaving a further crop of painful blisters. It's at this time that herpes is most likely to be transmitted sexually. It can take up to two weeks from the time the sores first appear until they finally go away. Some people never get another attack. Others get herpes again and again – often when they're run down or have another illness. Girls and women find that they frequently get a further attack when they're having a period. After the first one the attacks are usually a lot milder, and they often happen less and less often until they just stop happening altogether.

TREATMENT

There is no cure for herpes yet. Doctors can prescribe a medicine called Acyclovir which seems to help a lot with first attacks and some sufferers find it helps lessen the length of subsequent bouts. Otherwise, the following self-help methods may ease the discomfort:

—Take a mild painkiller.
—Wash the infected area with salty water, or put some salt into your bath.
—Wrap a few ice cubes in a clean bit of cloth and place on the sores.
—Keep the genital area cool; avoid hot baths.
—Apply a solution of witch hazel or surgical spirit to the sores.
—Wear cotton underwear, wear stockings, not tights, and avoid tight trousers.

PREVENTION

No kissing or oral sex if you or your partner has a cold sore. Definitely no oral sex or any type of sex which brings any part of your body in touch with the herpes sore. Make sure you wash your hands if you touch your genital herpes or cold sores. Don't use spit to wet contact lenses if you have cold sores.

LICE

Pubic lice, or crabs as they're commonly known, are unpleasant tiny creatures which like to live in the pubic hair
around the sex organs – but they can also get into the hair on
other parts of the body as well. They suck blood and lay their
eggs, called nits, that look like tiny white blobs at the hair
roots. You can catch crabs either by coming into close physical contact with someone who already has them, or from
bedding, sharing clothes, towels or even a toilet seat which
has just been used by someone with crabs. Whether your hair
is clean or dirty – crabs aren't fussy, they just want to
suck your blood and lay their eggs – they multiply quite
fast.

SYMPTOMS

They give you an itch which can almost drive you mad!

TREATMENT

You can't wash them away with ordinary shampoo – not even
medicated shampoo. You can buy a special lotion from the
chemist without a prescription. It is also available from a
special clinic. It usually takes about a week to get rid of
them.

PREVENTION

If you or your partner has genital lice don't have sex until you
are absolutely sure that every last creature and nit has gone.

MENSTRUAL PROBLEMS

Most women feel some pain or discomfort just before, during
or just after their periods. Pre-menstrual tension, or PMT as
it's known, is the feeling women get just before a period.
The pains are often much worse when a girl starts having
periods. The symptoms can include: stomach cramps, diarrhoea, constipation, swollen breasts, sore breasts, a general
all-over feeling of swollenness, a sudden bursting into tears

for no apparent reason, irritability, feverishness, a rise in temperature, or feeling low and depressed. The lucky ones feel nothing – or hardly anything – at all, while the very unlucky ones feel so bad that they have to take to their beds for a few days.

Many women suffer a great deal from some or all these pains and illnesses but put up with them because they think they're inevitable. They needn't be. There's absolutely no point in putting up with any pain that could be cured just because it's 'the time of the month'.

A painkilling pill can sometimes relieve some of the pain and discomfort. You can buy them from any chemist. A little extra light exercise can also help lessen the cramps. Many women find it helps to hold a hot water bottle to their stomachs or to have a bath.

If the pains get unbearable go to your doctor. Or if you find you're extremely tense just before a period, this can also be controlled by pills. Your doctor may be able to prescribe hormone pills which will regulate your periods and ease the pain. They may also make your periods much lighter. (These pills are in fact exactly the same as birth control pills, which can produce painful side-effects themselves. See page 107.)

Having a period doesn't – and shouldn't – mean that a girl has to stop doing anything she normally does. She can still go swimming (plunging into coldish water usually stops the flow for a while), wash her hair, play games, have hot baths and have sex if she wants to.

Don't be tempted to use your period as an excuse to get out of doing something – unless you feel really rotten. It makes people think that girls who do genuinely feel very bad are just pretending.

Some girls and women suffer from very irregular periods, known as dysmenorrhoea, and some from amenorrhoea, which means their periods stop altogether. When a girl's periods first start they are likely to be very irregular. But if they later become irregular or stop altogether, this is a sign that your doctor should investigate.

NON-SPECIFIC URETHRITIS
See under **Urethritis**.

NON-GONOCOCCAL URETHRITIS
See under **Urethritis**.

PELVIC INFLAMMATORY DISEASE
Often called PID for short. This is a serious disease for girls and women, usually caused by leaving other diseases like chlamydia and gonorrhoea untreated for too long. The inflammation and infection of PID spreads to the fallopian tubes and ovaries. The tubes become blocked and this may mean that she becomes infertile (i.e. is unable to have a baby).

SYMPTOMS
PID causes general feelings of being ill, tiredness, fever, pains in the lower part of the tummy and the back, an abnormal discharge, heavy or irregular periods, nausea and/or vomiting and pain during intercourse.

TREATMENT
Antibiotics taken by mouth can cure PID in its early stages. If left until very late, one or more of the infected internal organs may have to be removed by an operation in hospital. Women are usually so ill with PID that they'll probably have to stay in bed for a few weeks.

PREVENTION
Any abnormal discharge means that you should go to a special clinic for treatment straight away. The condom can prevent you from getting chlamydia or gonorrhoea in the first place.

PERIOD PAINS
See under **Menstrual problems**.

POST-GONOCOCCAL URETHRITIS

See under **Urethritis**.

SCABIES

The scabies itch is caused by a very tiny mite which burrows under the skin, particularly between the fingers and toes, the elbows, wrists and armpits, on the breasts and buttocks and occasionally in the genital region. They are transmitted by close physical contact and by dirty clothes, bedlinen and towels which contain the mites or their eggs.

SYMPTOMS

You can see their tiny black or white burrows just under the skin. Like lice, they are very itchy.

TREATMENT

Special lotions which you can buy from the chemist without prescription have to be applied to the infected areas.

PREVENTION

Clean clothing and regular baths are necessary to prevent re-infection. Don't have sex with an infected partner until all signs have gone.

SYPHILIS

Also known as the pox, this is a very serious venereal disease if left untreated. Sufferers used to die from it until penicillin was discovered this century. It can only be caught by anal or vaginal intercourse.

SYMPTOMS

The first symptoms appear three to six weeks after the infection has entered the body. They are the same for both females and males and pass through three different stages. During the first stage a painless sore which looks like a spot develops on or near the vagina or penis and occasionally around the anus or mouth. During the second stage a copper-coloured skin rash develops anywhere on the body and the sufferer gets flu-like symptoms. These symptoms eventually disappear and during the third stage nothing can be detected. But the disease is attacking every single organ in the body. If untreated it leads to paralysis, blindness, madness and eventually death.

TREATMENT

It's extremely rare for syphilis to reach the final stage these days. Most people with this disease usually have some other infection in the vagina or penis which has made them go to a special clinic. The clinic tests for syphilis automatically. It's extremely easy to cure with antibiotics.

PREVENTION

Safer sex – using a condom – prevents syphilis from being transmitted.

THRUSH

See under **Candida albicans**.

TRICHOMONIASIS

Also known as Trich or TV for short, this is a tiny microbe which can be found in both females and males. Infection can be transmitted either by sexual contact or very occasionally by splashes on toilet seats or by using towels or clothes of an infected person.

SYMPTOMS

There may be no symptoms at all. Or there may be a horrid-smelling, yellowish-green or greyish, thin, foamy discharge from the vagina or penis. The vagina, vulva or penis may look red and feel sore. There may be some pain when peeing. It is often accompanied by cystitis and/or by gonorrhoea in females.

TREATMENT

The clinic will prescribe a course of pills to take by mouth.

PREVENTION

To prevent transmission by sexual intercourse, the condom is the answer.

URETHRITIS

This is an inflammation that men get in the tube running from the bladder to the tip of the penis. It has many different names and any of the following may be used by doctors or in the special clinic:

—NSU: Non-Specific Urethritis
—NGU: Non-Gonococcal Urethritis
—PGU: Post-Gonococcal Urethritis.

All three terms are used to describe urethritis when the germ causing the infection hasn't been discovered by laboratory tests. NGU means that gonorrhoea is not the cause of the symptoms. PGU means that the infection has been found in a man who has recently been cured of gonorrhoea. It is possible that urethritis was caught at the same time as gonorrhoea, but it isn't cured by the same drugs. It isn't possible to discover urethritis until the gonorrhoea has been cured.

SYMPTOMS

Pain when peeing and a discharge which, if the infection gets really bad, may be flecked with blood.

TREATMENT

It's important that samples of the discharge from the penis are examined at the special clinic under a microscope and by laboratory tests so that hopefully the infection is accurately identified and the correct treatment is given. Penicillin, which is the usual treatment for gonorrhoea, does not cure NSU. Other antibiotics will be given.

WARTS

Genital warts are spread by anal or vaginal sexual intercourse or from fingers to the genitals. It is believed that in women and girls there may be some connection between genital warts and cervical cancer.

SYMPTOMS

In the moist areas of the genitals they tend to be reddish-pink, painless little cauliflower-like growths. They may be as small as a full-stop or as big as a thumb nail. If they're inside the vagina it may be impossible to see them. On dry skin, such as the outside of the penis, they tend to be smaller, harder and a bit greyish in colour. They usually appear between one to nine months after getting the infection.

TREATMENT

The special clinic will treat warts according to their size. They may be painted with a special lotion or cream. The larger ones have to be burnt or frozen off, or they may have to be cut out. This is a painless operation which only takes a minute or two. Girls or women who have had warts must have regular cervical smear tests once a year.

PREVENTION

You should have no sexual contact until the warts have been removed. Safer sex – using a condom – will help prevent the transmission of warts.

Useful Addresses
and Phone Numbers

The following organizations, addresses and phone numbers were all checked at the time this book went to the printers (Spring 1988), but it's possible that by the time you read this they will have moved. If you have any difficulty in getting hold of any of these organizations, either contact a similar-sounding one or ask your local Citizens Advice Bureau. If you want to write to any of these organizations send a stamped addressed envelope (sae).

GENERAL HELP AND ADVICE

BRITISH ASSOCIATION FOR COUNSELLING

37a Sheep Street, Rugby, Warwickshire CV21 3BX. Tel. 0788 78328.
Provides an up-to-date list of local counselling and advisory centres and individuals that can give you expert advice on problems such as sex, drugs, living accommodation and other matters. Send sae to above address.

CHILDREN'S LEGAL CENTRE

20 Compton Terrace, London N1 2UN. Tel. 01-359 6251.
Provides free legal advice to young people and those still in full-time education. All advice given is from the young person's point of view. Phone during office hours. Write in for free leaflets and booklist concerning your particular problem.

CITIZENS ADVICE BUREAU (CAB)

In most towns and cities. Look in the phone book and ring up to find out opening hours. Gives free and confidential advice on a wide range of subjects including legal aid, welfare benefits, how to fill in forms and where to go for other organizations which can help solve your problem. You can phone or go to any CAB, not just your local one.

CLAIMANTS UNION

Groups to advise you about receiving social security, unemployment benefit or other benefits. They fight for claims at social security offices, appeal to tribunals and in courts. Very clued up on what all our rights are. Ask your local CAB for your nearest group.

EQUAL OPPORTUNITIES COMMISSION (EOC)

Overseas House, Quay Street, Manchester M3 3HN. Tel. 061 833 9244.
Gives free advice, information and leaflets on all aspects of sexual equality.

LEGAL ACTION GROUP

242–244 Pentonville Road, London N1. Tel. 01-833 3931.
Will give you the address of your local Neighbourhood Law Centre and the name and address of a sympathetic solicitor in your area.

NATIONAL ASSOCIATION FOR YOUNG PEOPLE'S
COUNSELLING AND ADVISORY SERVICES

17–23 Albion Street, Leicester LE1 6GD. Tel. 0533 558763.
Write to them for the address of your nearest youth counselling service.

NATIONAL COUNCIL FOR CIVIL LIBERTIES (NCCL)

21 Tabard Street, London SE1 4LA. Tel. 01-403 3888.
A campaigning organization to safeguard our rights and freedoms. Provides a free and confidential information service on a wide range of subjects relating to your civil rights. Send sae for booklist.

NATIONAL COUNCIL FOR VOLUNTARY ORGANIZATIONS

26 Bedford Square, London WC1B 3HU. Tel. 01-636 4066
Will tell you about any organization that you need to contact to help with your particular problem.

NORTHERN IRELAND COUNCIL FOR VOLUNTARY ACTION

2 Annadale Avenue, Belfast. Tel. 0232 640011.
Same as above.

SAMARITANS

Branches all over the UK. Look them up in the phone book. Phone them if you want to talk to someone understanding about any problem. Helps the lonely, suicidal or despairing. You don't have to give your name or address. Phone lines are open twenty-four hours a day.

EDUCATION

ADVISORY CENTRE FOR EDUCATION (ACE)

18 Victoria Park Square, Bethnal Green, London E2 9PB. Tel. 01-980 4596. Mon.– Fri., 2 p.m.–5.30 p.m.
Will give you a run-down on your rights on all aspects of education, e.g. if you're pregnant and under school-leaving age, if you're expelled, if a teacher beats you (now illegal), etc. Information sheets available and booklets at varying prices.

DEPARTMENT OF EDUCATION AND SCIENCE

Elizabeth House, 39 York Road, London SE1 7PH. Tel. 01-934 9000. Ask for the Information Department. They'll tell you what your rights are under the various Education Acts. Several free leaflets.

AIDS

There are many organizations, helplines and advice centres you can go to or phone if you have any question about AIDS. The Terrence Higgins Trust (THT) is a really good place to phone or to contact for more information. But most towns and cities now have their own helplines. You can find out where your local centre is by phoning the Terrence Higgins Trust or your local special clinic (look it up in the phone book under Special Clinic or Genito-urinary Medicine Clinic, or ask the operator at your local hospital), or you can phone the National Advisory Service on AIDS. Here are some of the main AIDS helplines and organizations:

England

THE NATIONAL ADVISORY SERVICE ON AIDS

Freefone 0800 567 123.
A free 24-hour phone service which provides advice, counselling and

information if you have any worries about AIDS and would like to talk to someone in confidence. They also have a list of all the AIDS helplines throughout Great Britain.

TERRENCE HIGGINS TRUST (THT)

BM AIDS, London WC1N 3XX. (Admin.: 01-831 0330; Helpline: 01-242 1010; Vistel: 01-405 2463, 7 p.m.–10 p.m. daily, for the deaf and hard of hearing.)

Their helpline is open all week from 3 p.m. to 10 p.m. for advice, information and support for all those who have, think they may have, or know someone with AIDS or who are HIV positive. Caring, compassionate and very helpful charity organization. Send sae for leaflets. THT also runs a priority line for people with AIDS and those diagnosed antibody positive – the number can be obtained through hospitals and special clinics. THT also offers a number of support groups, services, etc. to people with AIDS, ARC or HIV infection. These include Body Positive, a self-help group for people who are antibody positive, a women's HIV/AIDS support group, a drug group, etc. Phone the Admin. number for details of these.

HEALTHLINE

Tel. 01-980 4848, 2 p.m. to 10 p.m.

Ask the Healthline operator to play tape number 228 which gives you a complete list of all the tapes they have about AIDS. For their tape 'AIDS and Young People', phone 01-981 7140 (local rates from London); 0345 581858 (local rates from outside London); or 0800 010 958 (free from anywhere in the UK).

Scotland

EDINBURGH SCOTTISH AIDS MONITOR

P.O. Box 169, Edinburgh EH1 3UU. Tel. 031 558 1167.

Lines open every evening from 7.30 p.m. to 10 p.m. Answerphone service at other times.

GLASGOW SCOTTISH AIDS MONITOR

P.O. Box 111, Glasgow G2 2UG. Tel. 041 221 7467.

Phone Tuesday, Wednesday, Thursday and Friday from 7 p.m. to 10 p.m. Answerphone service at other times.

Wales

CARDIFF AIDS HELPLINE
Tel. 0222 223443, weekdays from 7 p.m. to 10 p.m.

Northern Ireland

AIDS BELFAST
P.O. Box 206, Belfast, or offices at 310 Bryson House, Bedford Street, Belfast BT2. Tel. Belfast 326117.
Open Monday to Friday, 7.30 p.m. to 10.30 p.m.

Republic of Ireland

CAIRDE (FRIENDS)
10 Fownes Street, Dublin 2. Tel. Dublin 710939. Phone from Monday to Friday, 11 a.m. to 4 p.m.
A voluntary organization offering support and information on AIDS throughout the thirty-two counties. Although it's a part of the Gay Health Action group, it offers its services to anyone who feels they need help or advice, whether they're gay or not.

GAY HEALTH ACTION
P.O. Box 1890, Sheriff Street, Dublin 1. Tel. Dublin 788848.
Also has a Lesbian Health Action group. Provides information on AIDS prevention, sexually transmitted diseases and other aspects of gay health.

GENERAL HEALTH MATTERS

COMMUNITY HEALTH COUNCILS (CHC)
Look up your local CHC in your phone book, under Community Health Council. They can advise you on your medical rights, help you make a complaint and tell you where to go for advice on abortion, contraception, sexually transmitted diseases, drug problems, etc.

HAEMOPHILIA SOCIETY
123 Westminster Bridge Road, London SE1 7HR. Tel. 01-928 2020.
Offers information and advice for those with haemophilia, their

friends and relatives. Contact them for their book, leaflets, etc. on AIDS and haemophilia.

HEALTHLINE

Tel. 01-980 4848, 2 p.m. to 10 p.m.
This is the main switchboard number for a phone service that plays over 200 tapes about a wide range of different illnesses. An operator will ask you what tape you want to hear. If you're not quite sure, tell the operator what your problem is and they'll put on the tape you need. For most calls you pay local rates from anywhere in the UK; some are free.

HEALTH EDUCATION AUTHORITY

78 New Oxford Street, London WC1A 1AH. Tel. 01-631 0930.
Information and free leaflets on a wide range of health matters. Look up your local office in the phone book.

HERPES ASSOCIATION

41 North Road, London N7 9DP. Tel. 01-609 9061.
Offers an advice and counselling phone service. Ring the above number during the day and you'll be given the name and the number of the counsellor to phone during the afternoon and evening.

NATIONAL ASSOCIATION FOR PRE-MENSTRUAL SYNDROME

25 Market Street, Guildford, Surrey GU1 4LB. Tel. 0483 572 806.
For advice and counselling service, phone from Monday to Friday from 9.30 a.m. to 1 p.m., and from 9.30 a.m. to 12 p.m. on Tuesdays and Wednesdays. Evening line is on 09592 4371.

PATIENTS ASSOCIATION

Room 33, 18 Charing Cross Road, London WC2H 0HR. Tel. 01-240 0671.
A voluntary pressure group which advises patients of their rights and/or who want to make a complaint about any aspect of medical (mis)treatment or who don't know how to get medical treatment for some specific illness. Very helpful to young people. Free and confidential. Send sae for leaflets and publications list.

RELEASE

169 Commercial Street, London E1 6BW. Tel. 01-377 5905 (office hours); 01-603 8654 (24-hour helpline).

SPECIAL CLINICS

These clinics treat all sexually transmitted diseases. They're usually listed in local phone books under Venereal Disease, or VD, or Sexually Transmitted Disease, or Special Clinic, or Genito-urinary Clinic. You can phone your local hospital or doctor to find out where your nearest special clinic is.

WOMEN'S HEALTH INFORMATION CENTRE

52 Featherstone Street, London EC1Y 8RT. Tel. 01-251 6580.
Reference library of articles covering all subjects to do with women's health.

WOMEN'S NATIONAL CANCER CONTROL CAMPAIGN

1 South Audley Street, London W1Y 5DQ. Tel. 01-499 7532.
Provides information on cancer and how to get treatment. Has free leaflets, including some on how to check for breast cancer and what happens if you go for a smear test for cervical cancer.

SEX, CONTRACEPTION, PREGNANCY TESTING, ABORTION

ASSOCIATION TO AID THE SEXUAL AND PERSONAL
RELATIONSHIPS OF PEOPLE WITH A DISABILITY (SPOD)

286 Camden Road, London N7 9BJ. Tel. 01-607 8851.
Advice and information for anyone – or their relatives or friends – with a physical or mental disability. Send sae for leaflets and reading list.

BRITISH PREGNANCY ADVISORY SERVICE

Austy Manor, Wootton Wawen, Solihull, West Midlands B95 6BX. Tel. 05642 3225.
A non-profit-making charity. It has clinics in many towns and cities. Offers totally confidential and free pregnancy tests, sex counselling, birth control advice and supplies, pregnancy and abortion advice. Completely sympathetic to young people (boys and girls). Look it up in the phone book or contact above address for your nearest branch. If you need an abortion, the BPAS can arrange a loan and grant system for those who are hard up. Can arrange overnight and

outpatient abortions. Also very good for the disabled. Phone, write or call in. Very reasonable rates.

BROOK ADVISORY CENTRE

153a East Street, London SE17 2SD. Tel. 01-708 1234.
Also has centres in Birmingham, Bristol, Burnley, Coventry, Edinburgh, London and Liverpool. Gives confidential birth control advice and counselling to young people. Consultation and birth control supplies free at most centres. Fee charged for pregnancy testing and infection testing at some of the centres. Phone, write or call in. Very sympathetic to young people with little or no money.

FAMILY PLANNING ASSOCIATION (FPA)

27–35 Mortimer Street, London WIN 7RJ. Tel. 01-636 7866.
For your nearest FPA clinic, look it up in the phone book or contact the above address. Provides free and confidential advice and information to young people on birth control, abortion, sexual problems and sexually transmitted diseases, and a service of regular medical supervision, cervical smear testing and pregnancy testing. Issues a wide range of free leaflets on all these subjects. Has a fairly good booklist.

FAMILY PLANNING ASSOCIATION OF NORTHERN IRELAND

113 University Street, Belfast B7 1HP. Tel. Belfast 32488.
14 Magazine Street, Londonderry. Tel. Londonderry 260016.
You can go to any one of the fifty clinics in Northern Ireland, no matter where you live. They provide the same services as the FPA, above.

IRISH FAMILY PLANNING ASSOCIATION

15 Mountjoy Square, Dublin 1. Information centre: tel. Dublin 740723; Education resource centre: tel. Dublin 364533.
Clinics in Synge Street (tel. Dublin 682420) and Cathal Brugha Street (tel. Dublin 727276) provide a full range of birth control methods, help with sexual problems, a women's health service and pregnancy testing. Very helpful and sympathetic to women and girls with unwanted pregnancies. Fees according to how much you earn. Phone first for an appointment. The Synge Street Clinic runs a Young People's Family Planning Centre on Saturdays from 1 p.m. to 4 p.m. which offers 30 per cent discount for students and the unemployed under 23 and a free pregnancy testing service.

They also organize the ADOLESCENT CONFIDENTIAL TELEPHONE SERVICE, run by young people for young people, which offers advice and factual information on all sexual matters. This service can be phoned on Dublin 740723/744133/729574.

IRISH WOMEN'S ABORTION SUPPORT GROUP

Tel. 01-251 6332.
This group, based in London, can be contacted directly on Tuesdays from 6 p.m. to 9 p.m., or a message may be left during office hours. It arranges abortions in England for girls and women living in the Republic of Ireland and can provide accommodation (in London) when absolutely necessary.

NATIONAL MARRIAGE GUIDANCE COUNCIL

Herbert Gray College, Little Church Street, Rugby, Warwickshire CV21 3AP. Tel. 0788 73241.
An unfortunate name, as this organization runs clinics for couples over 16, married or not, who have sexual and relationship problems. Contact above address or look it up in the phone book for your nearest branch.

NEW GRAPEVINE

416 St John Street, London EC1V 4NJ. Drop-in and helpline: tel. 01-278 9147. Tuesday 10.30 a.m. to 2.30 p.m.; Wednesday 2.30 p.m. to 6.30 p.m.
A free sex education advice and information service for young people (under 25). Provides support and counselling for anyone with sex and personal problems. Will put you in touch with other helpful organizations.

PREGNANCY ADVISORY SERVICE

11–13 Charlotte Street, London W1P 1HD. Tel. 01-637 8962.
London-based registered charity providing much the same service as the British Pregnancy Advisory Service (see page 193).

ULSTER PREGNANCY ADVISORY ASSOCIATION LTD

719a Lisburn Road, Belfast BT9 7GU. Tel. Belfast 381345.
Has a free answering service. Counselling service for pregnant girls. Arranges abortions in England through the British Pregnancy Advisory Service (see page 193) and other organizations. Can provide an after-care service.

PREGNANCY, CHILDBIRTH, ADOPTION, FOSTERING AND PARENTHOOD

ALLY

Dominican Priory, Upper Dorset Street, Dublin 1. Tel. Dublin 732200.
Offers a sympathetic service for single pregnant girls. Runs a family placement scheme for girls to live with a friendly family while they're pregnant. Free after-care and advice.

BRITISH AGENCY FOR ADOPTION AND FOSTERING

11 Southwark Street, London SE1 1RQ. Tel. 01-407 8800.
Source of information and advice during pregnancy on the choice to be made between adoption and fostering. Send sae for free leaflets.

CATHOLIC PROTECTION AND RESCUE SOCIETY OF IRELAND

30 South Anne Street, Dublin 2. Tel. Dublin 779664.
Geared to help single pregnant girls. Can provide care for dependent babies in the form of temporary residential and short-term foster care. Can arrange adoptions. Free and confidential.

CHERISH

2 Lower Pembroke Street, Dublin 2. Tel. Dublin 682744.
Mainly for girls wanting to keep their babies, but also offers pregnancy counselling service, advice and accommodation during and after pregnancy.

GINGERBREAD

35 Wellington Street, London WC2E 7BN. Tel. 01-240 0953.
39 Hope Street, Glasgow G3 7DW. Tel. 041 248 6840.
171 University Street, Belfast BT7 1HR. Tel. Belfast 231417.
12 Wicklow Street (Top Floor), Dublin 2. Tel. Dublin 710291.
Self-help groups for one parent families, with over 300 branches throughout the UK. A small fee for joining. Send sae for publications list. Phone the nearest head office to find your local branch.

MATERNITY ALLIANCE

15 Britannia Street, London, WC1X 9JP. Tel. 01-837 1265.
Will give you advice on your rights, benefits and allowances during pregnancy and after the child is born.

NATIONAL CHILDBIRTH TRUST

9 Queensborough Terrace, London W2 3TB. Tel. 01-221 3833.
Offers friendly advice to pregnant girls and women about childbirth, being pregnant, breastfeeding, etc. Aims to take the fear out of childbirth. Encourages fathers to take part. Send sae for booklist, leaflets and details of nearest classes and charges.

NATIONAL COUNCIL FOR ONE PARENT FAMILIES

255 Kentish Town Road, London NW5 2LX. Tel. 01-267 1361.
Sympathetic, helpful and expert advice on all matters concerning single mothers and fathers. Offers advice without strings or pressures. Acts as a link between those who need information or advice and self-help organizations and groups, local social workers, and others who have the responsibility of providing services for one parent families and single pregnant girls. Inquiries dealt with by letter, phone or interview (best to book for appointment). Private and confidential. Will put you in touch with other useful organizations.

NATIONAL FOSTER CARE ASSOCIATION

1st Floor, Francis House, Francis Street, London SWIP IDE. Tel. 01-828 6266.
Information about having your child fostered.

PARENT TO PARENT INFORMATION ON ADOPTION SOCIETY

Lower Boddington, Daventry, Northants NN11 6YB. Tel. 0327 60295.
Write or phone for information and advice about adoption.

SCOTTISH COUNCIL FOR SINGLE PARENTS

13 Gayfield Square, Edinburgh EH1 3NX. Tel. 031 556 3899.
Friendly, sympathetic and helpful advice on all problems for lone parents and single pregnant girls. Free.

SINGLE HANDED LTD

Thorne House, Hankham Place, Stone Cross, Pevensey, East Sussex BN24 5ER. Tel. 0323 767507.
A registered charity which helps single parents find accommodation by introducing them to other single parents who want to share. Arranges group holidays for single parents.

SEXUAL ABUSE

CHILDLINE

Freepost 1111, London EC4B 4BB (no stamp needed). Tel. Freefone 0800 1111 (the number is the same wherever you live, and free).
A free 24-hour counselling and advice phoneline for children and young people in danger or in trouble – especially helpful to those who have been sexually abused and/or who want to run away from home. Totally confidential.

RAPE CRISIS CENTRE

P.O. Box 69, London WC1N 3XX. Tel. office hours: 01-278 3956; 24-hour emergency service: 01-837 1600.
For women and girls only. Look it up in the phone book for your local centre or phone above number for help. Provides moral support, legal and medical advice and counselling for girls and women who have been raped or sexually abused. Phone the emergency service number at any time, day or night, to talk with a woman who will be helpful, sympathetic and understanding. Most centres can arrange tests for pregnancy and sexually transmitted diseases and will find someone to go with you to the doctor or clinic, police station and court. Send sae to above address for more information about rape and sexual abuse.

INCEST CRISIS LINE

P.O. Box 32, Northolt, Middlesex UB5 4JG. Tel. 01-422 5100 or 890 4732.
Provides a 24-hour helpline, giving advice and practical assistance to those who have been sexually abused by a member of their own family or someone they trust. Phone them even if you're just scared that it might happen.

NATIONAL SOCIETY FOR THE PREVENTION OF CRUELTY TO CHILDREN (NSPCC)

67 Saffron Hill, London EC1 8RS. Tel. 01-242 1626.
Provides a 24-hour counselling and referral service. For local branches consult the phone book under NSPCC. Local branches also provide a 24-hour helpline.

·

SEXUAL IDENTITY

ALBANY TRUST

24 Chester Square, London SW1W 9HS. Tel. 01-730 5871.
Charitable organization concerned with educational research and the psycho-sexual health of gays, lesbians, bisexuals, transsexuals, transvestites and anyone with a sexual identity problem. Also a counselling service. Their phone line is open on Thursday afternoons to book an appointment and there is a 24-hour answerphone service. Send sae for booklist.

CAMPAIGN FOR HOMOSEXUAL EQUALITY (CHE)

Room 221, 38 Mount Pleasant, London WC1 0AT. Tel. 01-833 3912.
A campaigning lobby group for lesbians and gays. Campaigns for complete legal and social equality for lesbians and gays. Has some teaching resources. Contact for details of your local group. Open office hours.

CARAFRIEND

Tel. Belfast 222023; Londonderry 263120.
Phone lines are open Mondays, Tuesdays and Wednesdays from 7.30 p.m. to 10 p.m. Provides a befriending, information and counselling service for gays. Lesbian lines at Belfast and Londonderry are open on Thursday from 7.30 p.m. to 10 p.m.

GAY AND LESBIAN LEGAL ADVICE (GLAD)

69 Cowcross Street, London EC1M 6BP. Tel. 01-253 2043.
Free and confidential legal advice for lesbians and gays. Phone lines open Monday to Friday from 7 p.m. to 10 p.m.

LESBIAN AND GAY BLACK GROUP

BM Box 4390, London WC1N 3XX.
Send sae for details about groups near you.

LESBIAN AND GAY CHRISTIAN MOVEMENT

St Botolph's Church, Aldgate, London EC3N 1AB. Tel. 01-283 5165.
Has several groups around the country for lesbians and gays of all ages and of any Christian denomination. Send sae for further details.

LESBIAN AND GAY SWITCHBOARD

BM Switchboard, London WC1N 3XX. Tel. 01-837 7324.
24-hour phone and help service for lesbians and gays. Couldn't be
more helpful or friendly. A kind of lesbian and gay 'citizens advice
bureau', they provide information on all aspects of the lesbian and
gay world as well as running a flat-sharing service, dealing with
emotional problems, legal emergencies, chatting to the lonely and
counselling on AIDS. Will put you in touch with lesbian and gay
groups all over the country.

LESBIAN AND GAY YOUTH MOVEMENT

P.O. Box BMGYM, London WC1N 3XX. Tel. 01-317 9690.
Lines open Tuesdays, Wednesdays and Fridays from 6.30 p.m. to
8.30 p.m. For those under 26. Runs a national pen pal service. Phone
or send sae for more information.

LONDON LESBIAN AND GAY CENTRE

69 Cowcross Street, London EC1M 6BP. Tel. 01-608 1471.
Free counselling, café, discos, bars, exhibitions, bookshop, women-
only space, etc. Open midday to midnight on Sundays; 5.30 p.m. to
11.30 p.m. on Tuesdays, Wednesdays and Thursdays; 5.30 p.m. to 2
a.m. on Fridays; midday to 2 a.m. on Saturdays; shut on Mondays.
Very welcoming and friendly.

LONDON LESBIAN AND GAY TEENAGE GROUP

6/9 Manor Gardens, Holloway Road, London N7 6LA. Tel. 01-272
5741.
For 16- to 21-year-olds, a telephone advice service. Lines open on
Sundays from 3 p.m. to 7 p.m. and Wednesdays from 7 p.m. to 10
p.m. Also offers a counselling service on coming out and a meeting
place.

NORTHERN IRELAND GAY RIGHTS ASSOCIATION

P.O. Box 44, Belfast BT1 1SH.
Free help, friendly advice and information for gays.

PARENTS ENQUIRY

Rose Robertson, 16 Honley Road, Catford, London SE6 2HZ.
Tel. 01-698 1815.
Parents of lesbian and gay children will get extremely good and
comforting advice and information on what it means to be lesbian or

gay. Check with above address for addresses of groups in other towns.

QUEST

BM Box 2585, London WCIN 3XX. Tel. 01-373 7819.
Roman Catholic group for lesbians and gays of all ages. Phone line open Fridays, Saturdays and Sundays from 7 p.m. to 10 p.m.

SCOTTISH GAY SWITCHBOARD

P.O. Box 169, Edinburgh EHI 3UU. Tel. 031 556 4049.
Phoneline is open 7.30 p.m. to 10 p.m. every evening. Lesbian line: 031 557 0751, Mondays and Thursday from 7.30 p.m. to 10 p.m.; Bisexual line: 031 557 3620 on Thursday 7.30 p.m. to 9.30 p.m.
Has several branches in Scotland which provide information about social events of interest to sexual minorities, and a free legal advice service. Very helpful and friendly.

WOMEN

There are women's centres in many towns throughout the UK which provide a means for different groups and individual girls and women to get together. Some offer services such as pregnancy testing, advice on abortion, pregnancy, motherhood, lesbianism, etc. They welcome women of all ages and not just those who count themselves as being in the Women's Movement.

A WOMAN'S PLACE

Hungerford House, Victoria Embankment, London WC2N CPA.
Tel. 01-836 6081.
Open Tuesdays, Wednesdays and Thursdays from 1 p.m. to 7 p.m. A centre for meetings and information, with a bookshop. The best place to find out about women's groups in your area.

BELFAST WOMEN'S CENTRE FOR ADVICE AND INFORMATION

18 Donegal Street, Belfast BTI 2GP. Tel. Belfast 243363.
Information about the Women's Movement and local groups in Northern Ireland.

WOMEN'S CENTRE (SCOTLAND)

61a Broughton Street, Edinburgh EH1 3RJ. Tel. 031 557 3179.
Information about the Women's Movement and local groups in
Scotland.

WOMEN'S CENTRE (WALES)

58 Alexandra Road, Swansea. Tel. 0792 467365.
Information about the Women's Movement and local groups in
Wales.

WOMEN'S CENTRE (REPUBLIC OF IRELAND)

53 Dame Street, Dublin 2. Tel. Dublin 710088.
Information about the Women's Movement and local groups in the
Republic of Ireland.

Reading List

If you send an sae to most of the above organizations they will send you free or low-priced leaflets on the subjects they deal with. The following books will give you further information and many of them contain good lists of yet more books if you want to follow the subject up.

Carol Adams and Rae Laurikietis, *The Gender Trap*, Quartet, 1976. Book 1: *Education and Work*; Book 2: *Sex and Marriage*; Book 3: *Messages and Images*.

Enjoyable books about the sex roles imposed on young people in our society. Written for those at school, and for their teachers and parents. Each book has cartoons, poems, stories, extracts, interviews, questions and ideas for projects, discussion and debate.

Anna Coote and Tess Gill, *Women's Rights: A Practical Guide*, Penguin, 1981.

Everything you could want to know about women's rights in the fields of work, money, sex, marriage, divorce, separation, children, housing, consumerism, immigration, prison and the law, etc.

Anna Coote, Melissa Benn and Tess Gill, *The Rape Controversy*, National Council for Civil Liberties, 1986.

Low-priced pamphlet on the law, the myths, the facts, and on the changes that are needed in the law and in attitudes. Plus what to do if you are raped.

Alison Frater and Catherine Wright, *Coping with Abortion*, Chambers, 1986.

Clear, easy-to-understand guide to all problems related to having an abortion.

John Hart, *So You Think You're Attracted to the Same Sex?*, Penguin, 1984.

Clearly written, this book will reassure anyone who is worried about their sexual identity. Useful too for explaining that it's perfectly normal to be lesbian, gay or bisexual.

Suzie Hayman, *It's More Than Sex: A survival guide to the teenage years*, Wildwood House, 1986.

Clearly written and highly informative book on almost everything you could want to know about surviving.

Angela Kilmartin, *Understanding Cystitis: A complete self-help guide*, Century-Arrow, 1985.

Everything you need to know about this horrid illness – including lots on how to cope with it and prevent it.

Angela Phillips, *Your Body, Your Baby, Your Life*, Pandora Press, 1983.

One of the very best books about pregnancy and childbirth.

Angela Phillips and Jill Rakusen, *Our Bodies, Ourselves*, Penguin, 1978.

A lot of really valuable information on all aspects of women's health and sexuality, anatomy, relationships, exercise, health, sexually transmitted diseases, contraception, parenthood, childbirth, menopause, self-defence, rape, etc. Personal stories included.

Bill Stewart, *Sex and Spina Bifida*, ASBAH/SPOD.

Well-illustrated pamphlet specially for teenagers suffering from spina bifida and other related disabilities.

Rosemary Stones, *Too Close Encounters and What to Do About Them: A guide for teenagers*, Magnet, 1987.

This is a great book – really well written and wonderfully easy to read. All you need to know about every aspect of the misuses and abuses of sex. For girls and boys.

Peter Tatchell, *AIDS: A Guide to Survival*, GMP, 1986.

The best book for anyone who is HIV antibody positive or who has AIDS, and their friends, relatives and carers. It's very moving to read.

Ruth Thomson, *Have You Started Yet?*, Piccolo, 1980.

One of the best and easiest to read books written about periods for young teenagers (boys should read this too).

Lorraine Trenchard and Hugh Warren, *Something to Tell You*, London Gay Teenage Group, 1984.

You don't have to be a Londoner to enjoy and learn from this book of personal experiences of young lesbians and gays.

Index

FOR THE BEST IN PAPERBACKS, LOOK FOR THE

In every corner of the world, on every subject under the sun, Penguin represents quality and variety – the very best in publishing today.

For complete information about books available from Penguin – including Pelicans, Puffins, Peregrines and Penguin Classics – and how to order them, write to us at the appropriate address below. Please note that for copyright reasons the selection of books varies from country to country.

In the United Kingdom: For a complete list of books available from Penguin in the U.K., please write to *Dept E.P., Penguin Books Ltd, Harmondsworth, Middlesex, UB7 0DA*

In the United States: For a complete list of books available from Penguin in the U.S., please write to *Dept BA, Penguin, 299 Murray Hill Parkway, East Rutherford, New Jersey 07073*

In Canada: For a complete list of books available from Penguin in Canada, please write to *Penguin Books Canada Ltd, 2801 John Street, Markham, Ontario L3R 1B4*

In Australia: For a complete list of books available from Penguin in Australia, please write to the *Marketing Department, Penguin Books Australia Ltd, P.O. Box 257, Ringwood, Victoria 3134*

In New Zealand: For a complete list of books available from Penguin in New Zealand, please write to the *Marketing Department, Penguin Books (NZ) Ltd, Private Bag, Takapuna, Auckland 9*

In India: For a complete list of books available from Penguin, please write to *Penguin Overseas Ltd, 706 Eros Apartments, 56 Nehru Place, New Delhi, 110019*

In Holland: For a complete list of books available from Penguin in Holland, please write to *Penguin Books Nederland B.V., Postbus 195, NL–1380AD Weesp, Netherlands*

In Germany: For a complete list of books available from Penguin, please write to *Penguin Books Ltd, Friedrichstrasse 10 – 12, D–6000 Frankfurt Main 1, Federal Republic of Germany*

In Spain: For a complete list of books available from Penguin in Spain, please write to *Longman Penguin España, Calle San Nicolas 15, E–28013 Madrid, Spain*